### WHAT'S UP WITH . . .

Your period—is it as annoying as everyone says?
Your friends—what do you do when they're bad for
your health?
Diets—do any of them work? What else can you do to
stay in shape?
Your skin—how can you give zits the slip and keep
a healthy glow?
Romance—how do you know when you're ready for it?

### FIND OUT IN
### YOUR BODY: THE GIRLS' GUIDE

# Your Body

## the Girls' Guide

Janis Brody,
Ph.D.

St. Martin's Paperbacks

To my mother, Barbara Brody, who introduced me to my dance-skating groove and believed that I had the potential to be anything I wanted to be.

YOUR BODY: THE GIRLS' GUIDE

Copyright © 2000 by Janis Brody.

Illustrations copyright © 2000 by Deep Dutta.

ISBN: 0-312-97563-5

Printed in the United States of America

St. Martin's Paperbacks edition / August 2000

10  9  8  7  6  5  4  3  2  1

# Acknowledgments

I am tremendously grateful to so many generous people. Many, many thanks to my research assistants Ashley Novak, Liz Zach, Yun Xian Ho, Brad Reid, Melissa Rampy, Ariel Harman, and Joanna Lehman, who graciously offered their assistance above and beyond the call of duty. Thank you to Dr. Julie Jones and Sarah Warner who offered their expert consultation. I'm grateful to my girl reviewers, Elizabeth Fielder and Margot Bernstein, for their insight and encouragement. I'm beholden to my friends who generously provided their time and professional expertise: Dr. Judith Schteingart, Dr. Jill Putterman, Dr. Henry Kronengold, Cindy Summers, Dr. Shara Pulver Israel, Rachel Schwartz, Dr. Bonnie Sacks, Alice Stopkoski, Andrea Klausy, Mimi Dutta, Olugbemisola Amusa-Shonubi, Dr. Don Summers, Dr. Ellie Ehrenfeld, Sonya Lazarevic, Dr. Eva Moskowitz, Valery Simon, and Marc Weitz. Many thanks to Rose Greenberg, Gene Cohen, and John Watts for their unflagging friendship and support. I am indebted to Deep Dutta for producing outstanding original illustrations, and to my brother, Vic Brody, for connecting me to the Duttas. Thanks to my mother who provided storage space just at the point when my apartment was overflowing.

Many thanks to Joe Veltre, my editor at St. Martin's Press, for providing insightful feedback on the manuscript and for believing in the book. I'm very grateful to Christy Fletcher, my agent at Carlisle and Company, for her dedication to the book, and to her assistant Lori Applebaum for her editorial input. Thanks to Judy Blume for guiding me to my agent, and thanks to my grandmother, May Rubin, and Hilda Cooper for leading me to Judy Blume. Thanks to Julie Taylor for her generous career support, and to Health Education Services and ETR Associates for their educational material support. A special warm thanks to my cousin Nancy, who was my big sister advisor growing up, and to her children—Kara and Eliza Krakower—endless sources of girlpower inspiration. I send my appreciation out to my considerate neighbors in Route 66 and apartment #6, and to Al and everybody at the Bagel Zone. To the Central Park Dance Skaters Association and Leroy, the winter music man, many thanks—I could not have written this book without taking skate-dancing breaks.

The immense person-power behind this book is a tribute to how much people care about the future of girls.

# Contents

# Introduction
## The Secrets You Will Hear

As a girl today you're in the position to have it all; you can be both as feminine and as tough as you please. Taking the world by storm isn't always easy, especially if body blues are bringing you down. Did you know that girls are usually more self-confident than boys are until puberty hits? That when bodies begin to change, girls' confidence tends to spiral downward, while boys' self-assurance starts climbing high? Has this happened to anyone you know? Or to yourself?

There are girls who manage to resist the confidence tumble, and fortunately, I was one of them. It certainly wasn't because my body was perfect; my body wasn't growing upwards and outwards as I had hoped. But I didn't have time to worry about whether or not my breasts would grow bigger because I was absorbed in loving algebra, pondering my latest crush, and being amazed at how in ballet class I was able to lie down on my stomach, arch my back, and lift my toes all the way around to touch my chin. I perceived no limits on what my mind and body could do. In this book, I will help you feel the same.

I'm excited to share all of my resister secrets with you. Maybe you're already a resister whose self-esteem is flying high. If not, you can be. If your self-confidence has started to go underground, we can pull it right back up again. This book is designed to help you

- Love your body for all the amazing things it can do
- Be in fantastic shape simply by doing activities you love
- Be fit and trim by eating foods you adore and not counting a single calorie
- Eat nutritiously so that your skin glows, your mind soars, and your body blossoms
- Understand your body's changes and how you feel about them
- Hold on to good friends while sticking by the healthy choices you make
- Appreciate your body for the snowflake that it is—not for its fragility, but for its uniqueness

Quiz questions will help you assess areas in which you're strong, as well as where you may want a boost. The tips and actions are all about building your confidence so you can keep the body blues away. If you try an exercise and it doesn't work out, give yourself a break, and try another. Trying something new in your life is a lot like trying on clothes: Some may feel right, while others just aren't your style. If in this book I say something you disagree with, that's okay; thinking for yourself is what this book is all about.

Along with my resister secrets, I'll be sharing stories of my own body insecurities and how I triumphed over them. Sure, I'm a psychologist, but more important, I was once a girl, which means that I've been there too. If you like, just think of me as a big sister with a little extra wisdom.

This book is like a conversation between you and me. When I ask for your opinions or ideas, I mean it; I really want to hear what you have to say. You can let me know what's on your mind by visiting my Website, *TheGirls-Guides.com*. If you don't have Internet access at home or at school, your local public library might be a good way for you to surf the Net for free.

My hope is that after reading this book, body worries will be less of a drain on your brain, so that you'll have more thinking power. A wish of mine is that someday, at least one of you reading this book will be President of the United States—maybe it will be you. Turn the page and let the confidence-building begin. . . .

# ONE

## How You See Yourself— Loving Your Body

*Two girls have just gone shopping for summer clothes. They've returned home and are checking out their new looks in the mirror...*

Simone bought her new dress to wear to her best friend's birthday party. She's modeling the dress with her party shoes. It's not how the dress fits that she cares about; it's how well it flares out when she twirls. In front of the mirror, Simone twirls and twirls. "Yes! A great twirly skirt—just like Cinderella at the ball. I can't wait until the party." She stops and looks at herself, her face flushed red from spinning. "I look so pretty in this dress," she says to her reflection and runs off to the kitchen for a peanut butter and jelly sandwich.

*Kathleen is trying on the bathing suit she bought for summer camp.* "I look awful! My thighs are huge!" She turns sideways for a profile view. "My stomach is bulging—I look like I'm pregnant! At twelve! It's my breasts that I want to bulge, but it's more like, breasts, where are you? I'm never going swimming. I'll just say I have a stomachache, and sit on the side of the pool wearing a towel." She grabs a towel from the bathroom and returns to the mirror, checking out *her wraparound towel look. "I still look awful! Look at those fat thighs sticking out. Just forget the whole thing." She collapses on the bed in tears. "It's diet or die."*

Why did Simone enjoy her new dress, while Kathleen felt awful in her bathing suit? Kathleen is twelve years old, while Simone is eight. Simply being a preteen or teen girl these days makes you more vulnerable to feeling badly about your body. With your body and all your friends' bodies changing at different paces, boys coming onto the scene, and images of teen models everywhere, it's no wonder that loving your body becomes more and more of a challenge. How are you doing in the body-lovin' department? Are you holding on to those good feelings from when you were younger, or are they slipping away? This quiz will help you figure it out, and then—I promise I won't leave you hanging—an abundance of advice will follow on how to cherish your body.

> Researchers found that 60 percent of girls ages eight to nine have healthy self-esteem, but by high school, only 29 percent of girls are happy with themselves.

## Quiz:
## Do You Dig or Diss Your Bod?

For each question, please circle the *one* response that best fits how you feel about your body.

1. When I check myself out in the mirror, I think:
   a. Ugh! Look at my body; I'm *so* ugly!
   b. Why can't I look like someone else?
   c. I'm stylish, but my body could use a little work.
   d. I'm looking good.

2. When I meet another girl, the first thing I focus on is:
   a. How attractive she is compared to me.
   b. How attractive she is compared to the "beauty ideal."
   c. Her clothes and how they fit her.
   d. Her personality.

3. If people compliment my appearance, I think:
   a. They really think I'm ugly; they just don't want to hurt my feelings.
   b. They don't mean it; they're just trying to be nice.
   c. They say that to everybody.
   d. They're right.

4. When I meet new people, I'm sure they're thinking about:
   a. How ugly I am.
   b. What they like and don't like about my body.
   c. What they think about my personality.
   d. How much they like me all around.

5. The idea of plastic surgery to alter a part of my body:
   a. Is something I often think about doing.
   b. Crosses my mind from time to time.
   c. Is something I've never considered.
   d. Seems absurd—I like myself as I am: 100 percent natural!

6. When you ponder your life, you think:
   a. I'd be so much happier if I just had a different body.
   b. I wish my body didn't bring me down sometimes.
   c. I'd like to change a few things about my appearance, but overall I'm content.
   d. I'm happy being me.

7. Wearing a bathing suit in public:
   a. Is something I try to avoid at all costs.
   b. Makes me feel very self-conscious.

   c. Is not my favorite thing to do, but it's no big deal.
   d. Is something I enjoy.

8. When I'm doing a physical activity like a sport or dancing, I think:
   a. Everybody is staring at how ugly and awkward my body is.
   b. Everybody is staring at how uncoordinated my body is.
   c. How I wish my body were more coordinated.
   d. How I love the great things my body can do.

9. When I think about my body, I feel:
   a. Disgusted and want to cry.
   b. Embarrassed and want to hide what I don't like.
   c. Indifferent to how my body is shaped but happy with what it can do.
   d. Proud of my body's shape and abilities.

**Scoring the Quiz:** An (a) response = 1 point; (b) response = 2 points; (c) response = 3 points; and a (d) response = 4 points. If your total score falls between 29 and 36, then you're Diggin' Your Body; between 21 and 28, then you're Unsure About Your Body; and between 9 and 20, you're Dissin' Your Body.

**Diggin' Your Body:** Congratulations! You love your body and there is absolutely no shame in that. You also appreciate the importance of who you are on the inside. The trick for you will be to resist the pull to participate in body-bashing talk with the girls and to ignore advertisers' attempts to make you feel unattractive. This chapter will help you do just that. If you have any secret recipes for lovin' your body, please send them my way so I can pass them on to other girls through my website.

**Unsure About Your Body:** One day you like your body, the next day you don't. One day your body is your friend, the next it's your enemy. How you feel about your body is threatening to take over your self-image. You wish you could banish the bad body feelings because they take your energy away from enjoying friends, school, and activities. This chapter will help you do just that.

**Dissin' Your Body:** The body blues are getting the best of you and completely clouding your ability to appreciate your wonderful personality and the amazing things your body can do. It's time to fight back. You were born loving your body and all it could do for you, and somewhere along the way you learned to dislike yourself. Anything learned can be unlearned, and that's just what we'll work together to help you do.

Every girl was born preprogrammed to appreciate her body and all the new skills it can learn. Have you ever seen the gleeful look on a baby's face when she's just learned how to walk? That was you, too. Since you were designed to feel good about your body and all it can do, if you have the body blues, how did you catch them? We'll unravel the Mystery of the Bad Body Feelings, looking for clues in the media, your family, and your classmates. Like all good mysteries, this one will end with apprehending the culprits; you'll be able to take control and feel good about yourself.

---

Surveys have found that anywhere from 64 percent to 85 percent of American girls feel unhappy about their bodies—with the number of dissatisfied girls increasing rapidly throughout the teen years.

---

## The Beauty Trap

Picture all the girls in your math class. Do they all look alike? My guess is that their bodies come in quite an assortment of shapes and sizes: round, short, tall, big, petite, bony, fleshy. This is my guess because this is how girls are supposed to look. Yet most girls feel pressure to look like someone else, the *same* someone else—that someone else being the model on the cover of the latest magazine or the stick-thin actress on their favorite TV show. Many girls are thinking, "If only I could be tall, thin, big-breasted, and long-legged, I'd be popular and all my troubles would melt away."

Here's some astonishing news: Girls who most closely resemble the "body ideal" aren't necessarily happier than those who don't. In fact, they may even be more *unhappy*. Researchers have found that when people meet a female who appears to match the culture's current beauty ideal, they tend to assume that she has an unattractive personality; they think she's probably selfish or stuck-up. The "beauty ideal" girl often finds that other females don't want to be friends with her out of envy or mistrust. Did you ever wonder why many of the so-called "most beautiful" girls hang out together? The natural assumption would be that they were being snobby. But it's worth considering the possibility that they might think *you* don't want to be *their* friend.

> Very tall and very thin models represent only about six percent of all the body types of actual women.

## Beyond Body Esteem

So if girls who feel insecure about their bodies long to attain an "ideal," while the few girls born into the "ideal" aren't necessarily happy either, who's happy? The answer is those girls whose self-confidence is derived from many different areas of their lives. Self-esteem is made up of a number of components, **body esteem** being just one of them. Think of all the different esteems you have: There's intellectual esteem, creative esteem, athletic esteem, personality esteem, spiritual esteem, and relationship esteem. Do you realize that out of all these esteems, only the body esteem has a cultural standard that is impossible for more than 90 percent of us to achieve?

---

When junior high girls were asked what was the most important factor in their feeling good about themselves, what do you think they answered? The most common response was their looks.

---

I'm sure that in high school, my body esteem was high some days and lower on others, but I barely noticed the fluctuations because I had so many activities going on that something was bound to go my way on any given day. Maybe I didn't like the way I looked in my jeans, but I mastered a dance step; maybe I hated my haircut, but had a satisfying heart-to-heart with a friend; or maybe I noticed how short I was compared to my best friend, but sold my jewelry creations to a new store. What are the different areas of your life that give you an opportunity to feel good about yourself? To boost all of your esteems, try the following tips.

### ACTION: The Many Reasons to Admire Yourself

1. **Admiring Others.** Think of five people in your life whom you most admire. Write down the qualities about them that earned your respect and love. Looking at the list, do any of these characteristics have to do with appearance? My guess is not many do, if any at all.
2. **Admiring Yourself:**
a. **Reexamine the list, circling the characteristics that apply to you too.** I'm sure that you have several positive traits in common; we usually feel closest to

the people with whom we share certain positive characteristics.

b. **Come up with more.** On a separate sheet, write down the positive traits you circled that apply to you, and now add a few more. Think about the good things your favorite teacher or best friend would say about you. Don't be shy. Being able to think great thoughts about yourself is an important skill to master, and there are no limits.

c. **Ask a friend to help.** If you are really stumped, work with a close friend to jump-start your list. You could each write down why you like the other and then share what you wrote.

d. **Post it for inspiration.** Write each of your favorite positive self-descriptors on a different sticky note and stick them everywhere: on your mirror, inside a school notebook, next to your alarm clock—even use one as a bookmark.

3. **Know Thyself.** It's also good to be in touch with a few weaknesses that need development; not a single one of us is perfect. So make a list of the traits you would like to build up. An example of strength versus weakness for me would be: I come up with new creative ideas all the time, but I'm often too impatient to pursue them in depth.

4. **Explore Your Talents.** Find outlets for all the different types of self-esteem that you're not currently expressing. Maybe join a nature exploration club or a soccer league, volunteer at a nursing home or an animal shelter, take up painting or guitar, get a pen pal or join a girls' club. (See the website for ways to explore your potential.)

There was a popular belief in the late 1800s that the female frame was too fragile and weak to hold itself up. Women were encouraged to have a couple of ribs removed and then use corsets to keep their bodies straight.

# The Days When Thin Was Out And Plump Was In

Thin may be in now, but for most of history, Western civilization considered a plump female form to be the most attractive. Pleasantly plump was a sign that a woman was well-off and well-fed. Starting in the nineteenth century, women remained curvy, but were encouraged to squeeze in their flesh by wearing uncomfortable devices, such as corsets, which exaggerated their breasts, hips, and small waists. In the 1920s, the female fashion trend took a turn toward a youthful, independent look. (The fashion industry has to reinvent itself periodically in order to sell new clothing and stay in business.) Women cut their hair into short bobs and shortened their skirts; some even bound their chests with special flattening devices (Eek! Ouch!).

Full-figured women came back in vogue after World War II. Makes sense to me; at a time when the world is pulling out of a crisis, people want to be reassured with images of women who aren't starving to death. Then, starting in the 1960s, two opposing forces influenced how females felt about their bodies. The feminist movement was championing the glory of the variety of female forms. At the same time, fashion magazines started making a lot of money by presenting models with skinny, unattainable bodies. Although the feminists are still fighting the body acceptance battle, the media has been pushing the "thin is in" message to the max.

---

Who is considered the most popular sex symbol of all time? Marilyn Monroe, who was at her peak in the late 40s and early 50s. A full-figured woman, Marilyn Monroe was no size 6 (what size do you think she was?)—today she would be considered overweight and out of shape and probably be out of work.

# Today, Anorexic Thin Is In

Just a couple of years ago, the fashion model Kate Moss gained supermodel status with her anorexic, pre-pubescent-girl look; the trend caught on and controversy followed. Many of the leading actresses on today's most popular TV shows are suspected to be anorexic, including *Ally Mc-Beal*'s Calista Flockhart and *The Practice*'s Lara Flynn Boyle. If you're a fan of the show *Friends*, compare the new episodes to the old 1994 reruns and examine how much thinner the actresses have become, especially Courteney Cox Arquette and Jennifer Aniston. Also check out the male actors on the show; they've actually put on a little weight—which is what most people do naturally when they age.

Hollywood is wondering, "When will it end?" Kathy Najimy, co-star on the TV program *Veronica's Closet* said, "The glamorization of thinness is what's truly frightening, because if it continues, I really think we are going to see a woman drop dead on one of these television shows."[1] Americans are beginning to examine what it means when women who look so unhealthy are held up as the ideal. Today, I see small signs of a backlash brewing; in the media section I'll talk about these, along with ways you can join in the healthy body revolution.

In the scheme of history, it hasn't been very long since thin has been in. But from our short perspective, this period seems like an eternity, especially since the majority of us don't match the current "ideal." I wish I had the magical powers to recommend the following:

### ACTION: Time Travel—Visit a Historical Period When Your Body Type Was Revered

But since I'm but a mere mortal, I could recommend in its place that you travel to a different country or visit with people of different ethnic backgrounds in your own city or town.

It's not so much that females of different cultures have such different body types from each other. (In fact, there's a lot of variation within each cultural group.) It's that the American Caucasian culture gives the message that there's only one standard against which to measure beauty, while most other cultures embrace a wide variety of body types— in other words, they appreciate how girls and women actually look. This means that females of other cultural backgrounds may feel more comfortable and confident being themselves.

Some cultures encourage a plumper female form. A friend of mine heard Rosie O'Donnell tell the following story on TV: Rosie flew to a Latin country with a fashion model friend of hers. Upon arrival, the men admired plump Rosie, ignoring the model except to tell her that she needed to get some meat on her bones. Since you may not have easy access to other cultures, there's a simple solution— visit a museum.

### ACTION: Museum Mission

In past eras, when there were no televisions, billboards or fashion magazines, paintings and sculptures were the mediums for communicating current body trends.

1. **Grab a Buddy.** Take a friend, your mom, or your sister and head to the nearest museum that has European paintings from the nineteenth century and earlier. (If you can't find one close by, then go to a bookstore and thumb through the art books. On your next visit to a big city, pop into a museum.)

2. **Be on the Lookout.** Keep your eyes open for paintings that honor the beauty of fleshy young women with smallish breasts and ripples of thighs and buttocks. On my trip to the Metropolitan Museum of Art in New York City, I found paintings of plump nudes

by the Flemish Rubens, the Italian Titian, and the French Renoir.

3. **Take the Challenge.** I challenge you to find any paintings and sculptures of artwork from the nineteenth century and earlier that depict a tall slender woman with large breasts and small buttocks. During my two-hour tour of paintings and sculptures from all over the world, I was unable to find a single piece of artwork representing the current beauty ideal. If you find any in *your* museum of choice, go to my website *TheGirlsGuides.com* and let me know.

---

The ancient Greeks were so taken with the beauty of the female hips that they created a spectacular temple in honor of Aphrodite Kallipygos, the goddess with beautiful buttocks.

---

## The Media's Subliminal Seduction

Why do you think everyday "normal" looking women are the models in ads for everyday necessity products, such as cleaners, while "knockout" models are used to sell beauty products, like makeup? Since we need cleaners, but can survive without beauty aids, advertisers try to convince us that we must have these unnecessary products. The ad executives are counting on the fact that hardly any of us real females look like the models; the goal is to manipulate us into believing that if we only bought that specific brand of nail polish, we too could look like the "ideal" woman.

When selling kitchen products, the ads present women with whom we can identify; the goal is to make us female consumers think, "That woman looks like me. If she likes the product, then I'll probably like it too." (Why there aren't more males portrayed in cleaning situations is an important question, but a different book.)

The beauty companies spend a lot of money trying to get us females to chase after an illusion. An illusion, not just because nail polish isn't the key to attractiveness, but also because the models themselves don't really look like they appear in the ads. Did you know that many famous models and actresses walk through the streets unrecognized every day? Here are ten reasons why the mega media stars aren't really who they appear to be:

1. They are wearing a ton of makeup, even if they're simply trying to attain the "natural look."
2. The photographers use certain tricks with camera angles and lighting techniques to create "perfection."
3. The majority of model photos are retouched using special airbrush techniques or altered on a computer.
4. Many models have had at least one part of the body permanently altered through surgery.
5. Some models are anorexic—practically starving themselves to death to stay stick-thin.
6. Many live under the command of a whole army of personal dieticians, cooks, and personal trainers.
7. Many actors and models sign a contract that specifies their allowed weight.
8. Modeling agencies and fashion editors constantly weigh the models, pinch them, and scrutinize them from head to toe.
9. Some actresses are sewn into a rubberized body slimmer.
10. Sometimes when actresses' bodies are shown, it's really another woman serving as a body double.

It's genetically impossible for over 90 percent of women to make their bodies look like those of the fashion models and Miss Americas, no matter how much they're molded, starved, operated on, and made to work out.

The air of self-confidence that models present in ads is also an illusion. Most models are never satisfied with their own bodies; they constantly envy other models. Supermodel Cindy Crawford said that she was self-conscious about her arms and wanted Linda Evangelista's small arms. . . . Evangelista would like to be able to remove two of her own ribs and covets Christy Turlington's mouth. . . . Turlington hates her own feet and knees and thinks she has a beer belly.[2] The chain of envy never ends, even with models.

Is that why few models are smiling in photos—because they're unhappy with themselves? I think it's because the pout look is in. In my opinion, a smile beats a pout hands down. You smiling outshines a pouting model any day. You're probably thinking, "Only two people on earth would say that: you and my grandmother." No, really, beauty radiates when you smile, and when you laugh, watch out—beauty is everywhere. I'm not suggesting that you wear a fake smile. But I bet you didn't know that psychologists found that the act of simply smiling can make you happy; the smile muscles trigger the emotion. Try it now. Did it work?

> It takes the work of 43 muscles to make a frown, but only 17 to make a smile.

## The Healthy Body Revolution

Smiling and laughing are certainly two ways we can counter the model chic. In small ways, the media is beginning to help counter the beauty ideal as well. On TV, if you do enough channel surfing, you can find females who are much heavier than the usual super-slender models and actresses. There's the *Rosie O'Donnell Show*, *Veronica's Closet*, reruns of *Rosanne* and *Living Single*, and the actress Camryn Manheim on *The Practice*. Flip through the channels and if you find any other signs of revolution, please let me know.

> Comedienne and actress Janeane Garofalo, who looks like the typical woman, talks about her contribution to the body battle:
> *I have lost parts because of my size. I have made the decision not to go to the gym and hire a stylist, and it's cost me. But I've made that choice because I truly believe a woman's weight is a political issue, and if one young woman out there can see me and not feel crummy about herself, that's a good thing.*[3]

Teen magazines are starting to come around by publishing articles in which girls talk about why they enjoy their "non-ideal" bodies. For example, *Seventeen* magazine recently published an article entitled, "Not a size 6 and proud of it" (January 2000). While the teen magazines are making an effort to avoid dieting and body idealizing topics, beware of the women's magazines that still promote the body beautiful; this includes fitness magazines, which advance body obsession over health.

The way I look at it, we girls have two options. To put us on equal footing with the retouched fashion models, we could create a national network of videophones that runs everybody's images through a high-speed retouching computer, and then communicate using only these phones. Or we can be savvy media consumers who know when to fight back. I opt for the second recommendation. Maybe all of us together can turn the small amount of backlash into a full-scale revolution. Here are some ideas of where to begin.

> Research found that after only three minutes of looking at a fashion magazine, 70 percent of the women in the study felt depressed.

### ACTION: How to Manage the Media So That It Doesn't Manage You

1. **Analyze.** When you see an advertisement trying to sell the illusion of the ideal body, ask yourself, "Why does the advertiser want me to feel inadequate? What do they want me to believe their product will do for me?"

2. **Act.** After watching a TV program or movie, or reading a magazine, ask yourself how it made you feel about your body. If it made you feel insecure, determine why and:

   a. **Protest letter or E-mail.** Write a letter or E-mail directly to the TV station, the magazine, or the product company explaining your feelings. You just might find your letter published in the next issue of the magazine! Remember, you can get along perfectly well without these companies, but they need consumers like you in order to survive, so they want to hear what you have to say.

   b. **Girlcott.** Start a "girlcott" campaign against a company by drawing up a petition explaining your grievances along with a pledge not to purchase the product. Get people to sign it and then send the company a copy.

   c. **Alternative.** Choose an alternative TV show, a different publication, or a different activity altogether that doesn't involve the media, like playing a game with a friend or going for a bike ride.

3. **Positive Reinforcement.** If you felt happy and good about yourself after watching a show or reading a magazine: Let them know via mail or E-mail. I'm a strong believer in the power of positive reinforcement; this is when you increase the chances of something good reoccurring by saying, "That was great."

4. **Positive Female Role Models.** Decorate your room with posters of positive female role models, such as

athletes, writers, musicians, and women who helped make history.

5. **Influential Career.** Choose an influential career, such as a magazine editor, television producer, or fashion designer, and make it your mission to represent women and girls as we really are: unique.

---

In the U.S. over the last few decades, there's been increasing pressure to be thin. Miss America contestants have become slimmer, with smaller hips and breasts, while the average young woman between the ages of 17 and 24 has become heavier and heavier.

---

## Decoding Body Messages From Family and Friends

Your friends and family are steeped in media messages too; you all end up floating around together in a soup of insecurity. So, when you go to your mom, friend, or a sister for support in your struggles to feel good about your body, she might not be as reassuring as you need because she may have the same insecurities. And sometimes, someone you love may unintentionally wind up saying something that makes you feel worse. Instead of the blind leading the blind, it's the insecure leading the insecure.

### Your Mom

Moms have the tough job of trying to steer their daughters through the media maze and peer pressures, while coping with their own body issues. How do you think your mom feels about her body? Does she talk about calories or wanting to lose weight? Complain about the extra five pounds she put on over the holidays? Ask everybody how she looks? Or, does she float around the house at ease in her body?

Why so many questions about your mom? Poor body image is often passed down from mother to daughter. In all likelihood, you are built somewhat like your mom. In all likelihood, she wasn't helped to feel good about her body growing up. So she's bound to pass her bad feelings about herself on to you in some way, whether it's through less than flattering comments, hints that you should watch what you eat, or clothes-shopping guidance.

My mom, wanting what she thought was best for me, suggested that I "disguise" my "flaws" by wearing padded bras; the unintended message being that I wasn't good enough the way I was. I gave in to buying the bras, but they always sat at the bottom of my dresser drawer—I wanted to be me and be okay with that. I always wondered why my mom didn't know how beautiful she was.

When moms feel good about themselves, they have the power to make their daughters feel like queens. Raina, a successful larger-size model, was teased as a child for her size. But at home, her mother, who had a similar large build, always told Raina that "having a womanly body was something to be proud of."[4] Is it any surprise then that Raina grew into a woman eager to show the world her beauty?

---

Some fashion designers are taking advantage of women's weight concerns by relabeling their clothing with smaller sizes. The industry figures that a woman will be more likely to buy a piece of clothing that says that she's a size 6 over one that says she's a size 10.

---

## Your Dad

What's important to remember about dads is that your budding young womanhood may be awkward for them at first.

They just need a little transition time to work out new, but equally loving, ways to relate to you. Maybe that big bear hug is turning into an adoring shoulder squeeze. If he makes unflattering references to your appearance, let him know that his statements hurt your feelings, even if he is just joking. But also attribute the comments to his new-found awkwardness; he'll grow out of it eventually.

Since female bodies are a delicate matter, dads have a delicate balance to find. If he praises your appearance too much, you might mistakenly think that your mind doesn't matter. If he praises your mind, then you might mistakenly worry that he thinks you're ugly. I was lucky that my dad found the perfect solution; every time he complimented my appearance, he'd also say, "You're beautiful on the inside and outside." Most dads feel this way about their daughters, even though they're not necessarily able to express it outright.

## Your Friends

What do you and your friends talk about most? Your favorite music and TV shows? School? Boys? Or appearances? When you all talk about clothing, hair, and bodies, are the comments usually upbeat like, "Where did you get your hair cut? I love it," or downbeat like, "Doesn't this dress make me look fat? I've got to lose weight!"

Many of your friends may already be swimming around in the insecurity soup, and this can be enough to pull you in. Hearing a friend put herself down, when you think she looks great, can make you question your own self-confidence. Plus, everybody else's body-bashing can pressure you to feel as if you have to join in. You can find yourself in a Catch-22 situation: On the one hand, you worry about not having the perfect body. But on the other hand, you worry that you will be shunned if you actually like your body.

If a girl actually puts you down, remember that it might

be because she feels insecure about herself; misery loves company. "But she seems pretty high and mighty to me," you might say. Exactly—arrogance is a cover-up for insecurities. Anybody who is genuinely self-confident doesn't need to put somebody else down in order to raise herself up. If I had to boil down all my ideas about human relationships into one theory, I would call it the "Insecurity Is the Root of All Evil" theory. Any time relationships seem to go badly, impose my theory and let me know if it fits. Also remember that nobody in your life should be allowed to criticize your body, whether it be a parent, a girlfriend, a boyfriend, a teacher—anybody.

---

Eighty percent of seventeen-year-olds who are at a healthy weight see themselves as fat.

---

Here are a few suggestions on how to have positive body experiences:

### ACTION: Hushing the Critical Voices of Others

1. **Go Beyond Body.** If the people around you are bashing their own bodies, subtly try to suggest other topics of conversation or group activities. If they can't get a grip, tell them you think they're beautiful, this topic is driving you crazy, and you'd like to see if together you can all do something more productive.
2. **Choose a Strategy for Handling Criticism.**
a. **Give them the benefit of the doubt.** Assume it's their insecurities talking.
b. **Make them your ally.** Tell them you've noticed that a lot of girls and women have poor body images— even models. Then ask them whether or not they've ever been insecure. If so, how have they coped? Can they offer you any advice? You can show each other

photos and talk about how you felt about your bodies at different ages.

c. **Just say, "Yes."** One day I was walking to high school when a group of girls from a different school surrounded me, saying, "Look at how *short* you are." As if I didn't know this already. So I replied, "Yeah, I know." They laughed. I laughed. And we spent the rest of the way chitchatting. If somebody teases you about something that doesn't cut too deep, then just say, "Yes, you're right." This will probably leave them speechless; they'll likely change the subject or leave.

d. **Stand up to them or walk away.** If those girls had said, "Hello, little Miss Flat-Chested," I certainly would have felt too hurt to agree with them. So what could I have done? Walking away is always an option. Sometimes you might want to say simply, "Give me a break," along with one of those puzzled looks that communicates, "What's *your* problem?" It's not easy to come up with a quick response, especially when you're feeling wounded. Do whatever feels right to you in the moment, and remember that these people have some problems to work through.

3. **Promote a Culture of Compliments.** If a nice thought pops into your head about somebody's personality or appearance, say it out loud. Spontaneous compliments are great because people aren't expecting them. Your friends may act as if they don't accept the compliments, but deep inside it will warm their hearts—I promise. It certainly can be frustrating when a friend feels bad about her body and nothing you say seems to make a difference. Take comfort in the fact that the simple act of being her devoted friend helps her feel worthwhile, and maybe buy her a girl-power guide like this one. What you can do is be a good role model—accept compliments when they come your way.

# When You Talk to Yourself, What Do You Say?

Whether your ideas about your body originated in the media or friends or family, who is the worst culprit in the body battle right now? YOU! You have the ability, no matter how hard it might be, to recognize negative messages for what they are and toss them aside. Do you criticize yourself every time you look in the mirror, put on clothes, or walk around school? Then it's that tape playing in your head on perpetual rewind, saying, "I'm ugly."

A girl who has the "I'm ugly" tape going through her head is more likely to slouch and slink through the school halls. As a result, people will notice her less; not because of how she looks, but because she's trying to do a disappearing act and it works. Take the girls in my junior high school: Sarah was the most popular girl, so you might assume she was also the prettiest. The fact is that other girls were just as pretty, but what set Sarah apart was her self-confidence. She had two popular older sisters in the same school, so everybody knew her. It's great to feel good about yourself. There's no reason why you can't feel confident too.

The last action in this chapter is the hardest and the most important: learning to compliment yourself.

### ACTION: Replacing Criticisms with Compliments

1. **Write Down at Least Ten Compliments You Can Give to Your Body.** Contemplate each part of your body from the tippy-top of your head down to your little toenail. I counted more than 30 body parts, including eyebrows, smile, ears, shoulders, fingers, belly button, calves, and ankles. Plus, each body part has different features, like how your hair has texture

and color. If you didn't reach the goal of ten compliments, including at least one or two between your neck and knees, try to add to the list when you're in a different mood. Keep the list handy for a pep read when you need it.

2. **Rethink Your Insecurities.** When thinking about your body, were there any features that made you think, "No way can I find a compliment for *that*"? If so, answer the following questions for each trouble spot:

a. **What great action does this part of my body enable me to do?** There are arms for hugging, lips for singing, ears for listening to music, and hips for swaying to the beat. You get the idea.

b. **Why does this part of my body appear as it does?** Did I build up certain muscles from sports, get hips with puberty, inherit my Mom's feet, etc. . . .

c. **Where did I get the idea that this part of my body was inadequate?** Does my mom feel insecure about this part of her body? Did my brother make an offhand teasing comment just to get me going? Was I comparing myself to that actress on TV? And so on.

d. **Think of a comforting counterthought.** "I'm still growing," or "If I were in Spain right now, I would love my body." You see what I mean.

3. **Be on Criticism Alert.** If you catch yourself dissin' your body,

a. **First, apologize to yourself.** I'm serious—whenever I say anything to myself that's less than nice, I apologize and promise to try not to do it again.

b. **Second, ask yourself these questions.** "Would I say the same thing to a friend—and if I did, would I have any friends left?"

c. **Third, replace the criticism with a compliment.** After this exercise, you should have a bunch from which to choose.

d. **Fourth, remember that hushing your own critical voice can take time.**

Here are some big facts about small parts of your body:
One quarter of the 208 bones in your body can be found in
your feet; just one square inch of the skin on your hand
contains approximately 72 feet of nerve fiber.

## Mystery Solved?

So, were you able to solve the Mystery of the Bad Body
Feelings? Were any culprits apprehended and disarmed? If
after reading this book and trying the actions, you find that
dissatisfaction with your body won't stop plaguing you,
consider talking with a counselor. For guidance on how to
find an adult to talk to, see the chapter on Seeking Help,
pp. 248–249. Stop these destructive feelings now and save
yourself years of potential misery and body obsession.

During junior high and high school, I had a great way
of fighting off the body blues; I danced, whether in ballet
class, on roller skates, or in high school plays. Rather than
examine myself from the outside looking in, I lived inside
my body and enjoyed learning what it could do. Throughout my life, the times when I've felt the best about my
body are when I've been the most active. You too can discover the body beautiful by learning what makes your body
and soul tick. Chapter 4 will help you find your sports
groove.

Another great way to fend off bad body feelings is to know
what changes will be happening to your body during puberty and why. Read on. . . .

# Check Out These Resources

## Phone Numbers and Websites

National Association to Advance Fat Acceptance (NAAFA)
(800) 442-1214 (Recorded membership information) or
(916) 558-6880 (To talk with somebody weekdays.)
Website: *http://www.naafa.org*
Their goal is to end discrimination and empower fat people
through education, advocacy, and member support.

*http://www.melpomene.com*: A positive sports and body site
for girls and women.

*Teen Voices: The Magazine By, For, and About Teenage
and Young Adult Women*
(888) 882-8336 (Get information on ordering the magazine,
writing articles, or joining their peer mentorship and
leadership programs.)
Website: *http://www.TeenVoices.com*
The articles are written by teens, and the cover shows real
girls, not models!

General crisis counseling: Kid Save Hotline: 1 (800) 543-
7283 or National Runaway Switchboard 1 (800) 621-
4000.

## Books

Cooke, Kaz. *Real Gorgeous: The Truth About Body and
Beauty.* New York: W. W. Norton, 1996.
Douglas, Susan J. *Where the Girls Are: Growing Up Fe-
male with the Mass Media.* New York: Random House,
1994.
Ignoffo, Matthew, Ph.D. *Everything You Need to Know*

*About Self-Confidence.* New York: Rosen Publishing
   Group, 1996.
Manheim, Camryn. *Wake Up, I'm Fat!* New York: Broad-
   way Books, 1999.
Wolf, Naomi. *The Beauty Myth.* New York: Anchor, 1992.

## Movies

*The Truth About Cats and Dogs.* Dir. Michael Lehmann.
   Starring Janeane Garofalo and Uma Thurman (PG-13)

# TWO

# Puberty's Changes—Periods, Breasts, and More

In junior high school, a bunch of us were waiting at the bus stop, when Noah asked such a startling question that we let the bus pass us by. Noah had asked, "What's a period?" Well, we all knew enough to know that he wasn't asking about punctuation. We looked at our sneakers, picked at our fingernails, fiddled with our coat zippers, anything not to catch Noah's questioning glance. We were silent.

Rachel broke the silence, "Well, it's like there's garbage inside of you and it comes out." We crinkled our noses.

"That's gross," someone said.

Diane offered another idea, "It's like a nosebleed, except your you-know-what is bleeding." "Your what?" "What's a 'you-know-what'?" the boys asked teasingly until Diane said, "Vagina." People weren't pleased with this answer either. Nobody wanted a nosebleed.

Then I offered my theory, "It's like peeing, except blood comes out." At least my answer didn't gross them out too much, so they accepted it as the truth. But none of us really knew anything for sure.

You'll be happy to know that not one of those answers is right. There's no garbage and no steady stream like when you pee. The actual period process is gentle and natural, as are all the other changes that happen to your body on the inside and outside. Has your body started to change yet, budding breasts and sprouting hair in places other than the top of your head? Have you gotten "it" (your period) yet? All the changes that puberty brings can seem both thrilling and scary. Knowing what to expect can help turn fear into excited anticipation. How are you feeling about current and future body developments? Take the quiz to find out.

## Quiz:
### Body Changes—Arrive Today or Stay Away?

1. A woman's body is:
   a. Something I want to have because it's incredibly beautiful.
   b. Nothing special.
   c. Quite unattractive; I'd rather keep the body I have now forever.

2. When I think about having or getting my period, I feel mostly:
   a. Tingly all over.
   b. What's the big deal?
   c. Whoa, that's scary!

3. I hope that the changes to my body will:
   a. Happen A.S.A.P.
   b. Come whenever; I'm in no rush.
   c. Stay away for as long as possible.

4. When I think about growing breasts:
   a. I can't wait for them to grow to their full size.
   b. It doesn't matter much to me whether they come sooner or later.
   c. I worry that if they grow too big too soon, I'll feel self-conscious.

5. Having a womanly figure will signal to the world that I'm:
   a. Becoming grown-up and mature.
   b. Still the same old me.
   c. Wanting to have sex.

6. When the changes happen to my body, my classmates will probably:
   a. Be supportive in a smile-and-pat-on-the-back kind of way.
   b. Not really notice or pay much attention.
   c. Tease me and get on my case.

7. Pubic hair and underarm hair:
   a. Are signs of maturity.
   b. Don't deserve much thought.
   c. Seem undesirable and unattractive to me.

8. The changes that will or have happened to my body are something:
   a. I want the world to notice.
   b. I don't care whether people notice or not.
   c. I want to hide underneath clothing.

**Scoring the Quiz:** An (a) response = 1 point; (b) response = 2 points; and a (c) response = 3 points. When you add up your total for the quiz, if your score falls between 8 and 13, then you're **Excited** about puberty; between 14 and 18, then you're **Neutral**; and 19 to 24 means you're **Nervous**.

**Excited:** If you're totally bubbling over with excitement, that's terrific. You're happy being a girl and proud to embark on the journey of becoming a woman. Sometimes you may find yourself so eager to experience womanly changes, that you're disappointed when another girl changes in ways you do not. In this chapter, I'll be talking about how to predict when your body will change and how to avoid comparing yourself to others.

**Neutral:** If you're feeling blasé about the whole puberty thing, then this probably means that your thoughts are elsewhere, maybe on a special activity, school work, or the great feeling you get hanging with friends. Don't worry. Puberty will find you (if it hasn't already), you don't have to find it. Just continue enjoying your life and when you read this section, file the information away in the "save for later" folder in your brain.

**Nervous:** You should know that it's perfectly normal to be nervous about something unfamiliar that you know is coming but don't know precisely when. I'm happy to tell you that no matter how quickly or slowly your body changes, you will still be you. This chapter should help quell some of your fears by letting you in on what happens to your body during puberty. Sometimes girls are extra anxious because they've had a bad experience or gotten strong negative messages about becoming a woman. If this rings true for you, I will definitely address this issue later in the book. A growing girl is beautiful and should be free to feel in control of her body and have others respect it.

All this talk about puberty—what is it exactly? This is when your biological clock signals that it's time for your body to develop in ways that will make it possible for you to conceive, give birth to, and care for a baby. Your body goes through many different changes to reach its goal. Some changes you can see with your own eyes, while others remain hidden inside you. I'll discuss when and why breasts, pubic hair, hips, and more appear. Then we're in for some "period" talk.

## Body Changes You Can See With Your Own Eyes

Your body will be changing shape and sprouting hair in all sorts of places for several years, starting around age ten and continuing all the way through the beginning of college. The average age may vary depending upon your ethnicity. African-American girls tend to start developing a little earlier than Caucasian girls do, while Asian girls may begin a little later. I couldn't find any research on girls of other ethnic backgrounds, including Latin-Americans. Maybe you'll become a researcher some day and fill in the gaps in our knowledge.

Your genes do all the developing work; they have the program—much like a computer chip—to tell your body how tall you'll grow, how wide your hips will be, and so on. Your job is simply to take good care of yourself and watch your body's transformation with appreciation and awe. Typically breasts bud first, followed by body hair, and then hips, but every girl's maturation is unique in some way. Here's what to be on the lookout for.

## Breasts

**Breasts** develop through several stages, the first being the "breast buds," small round bumps that appear around age ten. The budding age varies widely—you may start at age sixteen while your friend may have already started at age eight. The breasts develop in stages; some girls' bodies rush through the different phases, while others take their sweet time. Starting age and blossoming rate have nothing whatsoever to do with the breasts' eventual shape and size. For a preview of how your breasts might look eventually, check out your mom's. Breasts and nipples come in a wide variety of shapes and sizes.

While your breasts are blossoming, your nipples are popping up, surrounded by a darker area called the **areola.** (I love the word "areola"—it reminds me of an angel's halo.) Sometimes nipples will stay pushed in. If this happens, don't worry, your breasts will still be able to do everything they were designed to do: produce milk and feed it to the young. That's what breast development is all about—the maturing of the milk ducts. And don't fret—you won't all of a sudden turn into a milk fountain one day; it takes pregnancy and children to set your breast-feeding system in motion.

---

Why do human females have two breasts with nipples, while female naked mole rats have 11? Because the maximum number of children that a woman is likely to give birth to is two, while the maximum litter size for the mole rat is 11. Just imagine what we would look like if triplets were common. How about a three-breasted bra?

---

If you discover that one breast is growing faster than the other, don't freak: That's also normal, and usually temporary. You're probably the only person who'll even notice—other people can't tell the difference. Sometimes adults say, "Girl, you're busting out," or "Hey, you're popping out." Don't worry, your breasts will not burst like balloons; these are just figures of speech.

**Bras.** In our culture, we can't talk about breasts without talking about bras. When should you start wearing one? Whenever you want. Some girls start when they get breast buds, some start before the budding begins, some wait until their breasts get big and uncomfortably jiggly, and others never start. It's all a matter of personal preference.

In my bunk at summer camp when I was 12, it was all about bras, not breasts. Bras were in; I was without, so I was out too. I coped by putting my energies into the softball team and horseback riding. Back at home, I bought a couple of bras, but hardly ever wore them. Even today, I only wear a bra when my clothes would be too revealing—no nipples shining through for me, thank you. My small, perky breasts are self-sufficient in the support department. If you develop large breasts, a bra can help keep you comfortable.

Bras may be common in America, but they are not the norm in all parts of the world. In parts of Africa, for instance, women rarely wear bras, so elongated breasts that droop way down are the style.

### ACTION: Bra Shopping

1. **Grab a Pal.** Feel free to ask your mom, big sister, or friend to go bra shopping with you.
2. **Training Bras.** Often when a girl is beginning to develop, she buys a training bra. Training bras come in all different sizes and styles, including sports bras. To find them, go to the girls' department.
3. **Regular Bras.** To buy a regular bra, you can go to the lingerie department and ask a sales lady to measure your bra size for a custom fit. A typical first bra is size 32AA. The "32" stands for the number of inches around a girl's body, right under her breasts, and the "AA" represents the smallest cup size. Cup size can range from AA, to A, B, C, and all the way up to D.
4. **Choosing One You Like.** Bras may be lacy, frilly or plain, and have an underwire or no wire. Some bras are padded to enhance the appearance of breast size, while some are designed to make breasts look smaller. My hope is that by the time you've finished reading this book, you'll prefer a bra that doesn't alter the appearance of your breasts because you will love your body. But it's OK to wear an enhancer or minimizer, especially if it makes you feel better.

## Body Hair

**Pubic hair,** which appears around the age of ten and a half, earned its name because it covers the pubic bone region.

The first hairs are like duckling fuzz—light-colored and soft. Gradually, they grow out in the shape of an upside down triangle and tend to become curly. The color may end up matching the color of the hair on your head, but the texture usually won't.

Why do you grow a garden patch of hair down there? Here's a clue in an analogy: Pubic hair is to vagina as eyelashes are to eyes. As puberty begins, your vaginal area becomes more sensitive to intruding microorganisms, such as germs, and pubic hair keeps them away, just like eyelashes prevent dirt from getting into your eyes.

> "Oh, my! My vagina is sweating!" True, this could happen to you—there are sweat glands in the vaginal area and they become more active during puberty. Deodorant sprays aren't recommended; just shower as usual and wear cotton undies—they're breathable and allow moisture to evaporate.

**Underarm hair** starts to sprout up around age 14. I bet that if I gave you 100 guesses as to why we develop underarm hair, you would still never get it. It's not that I don't think you're smart, I do. It's because I never would have guessed right either. Take a shot at it now; cover up the following paragraph and then think of as many different possible reasons as you can.

Okay, here's the answer: The reigning theory holds that armpit hair evolved in order to enhance the body odor (B.O.) produced by the sweat glands. B.O. used to be a powerful sexual signal to members of the opposite sex. In today's society, we've chosen to cover up our B.O. with deodorants and send other types of sexual signals.

> In many parts of the world, people don't feel the need to cover up their natural scent.

It should be no surprise, then, to hear that B.O. and underarm hair arrive at close to the same time. Before then, just washing regularly and wearing clean clothes should keep you smelling fresh. If you're unsure of your own B.O. status, dip your nose down and give yourself a sniff; believe me, you'll know if you catch a whiff. Have B.O.? Join the club. The action below will have you smelling sweet in no time.

**Other hair happenings** will be going on around your body. The hair on your arms and legs will probably feel thicker and get darker, especially for Caucasians, and generally less so for Asians. Variation among girls is great. Don't be surprised if a little hair appears around your nipples and belly button—this too is normal. Think of body hair as decoration highlighting your body features.

Contemplating taking the hair off your body as fast as it appears? Whoa! Wait a minute. Models and actors lack body hair, not because they come from a different species of human, but because they spend a zillion dollars on hair removal. Some Americans and other entire cultures elevate body hair to beauty heights. The Action will have a few tips.

### ACTION: Hair and Odor Control

1. **Masking B.O.** There are deodorants, which are like perfume for the pits; and antiperspirants, which dry up the sweat. These products come in every form imaginable: sprays, creams, sticks and roll-ons, and in scented and unscented varieties (I have yet to figure out how an unscented perfume for the pits works, but it does, so why question it?). Try a bunch of different kinds until you find the one you like best.

2. **Pubic Hair Belongs Down There.** I strongly advise not to go plucking or shaving your protective patch. First of all, ouch!!! Second, it'll itch like crazy!! Thirdly, it has a job to do—keeping you safe from germs. If you're upset that it seems unruly (even though it's supposed to be), then try a little careful trimming with very small manicure scissors.

### 3. Other Hair Removal.

**a. Hold off as long as you can.** Shaving takes regular hair maintenance because the hair always grows back. Waxing involves having hot wax poured on your skin, leaving it to dry and then ripping it off you, taking the hair with it. Sound painful? It is! There are other methods, such as electrolysis, which involve regular office visits and shelling out the bucks.

**b. If you're going for it**, start with the simplest methods: shaving or a depilatory (hair removing) cream. Find an experienced female to be your guide. If you fall in love with the hairless look, then consider the more elaborate means.

## The Oilies

**Acne** is elusive; it may appear as the first sign of puberty, the last sign or, if you're lucky, not at all. The puberty connection is that the hormones that stir your reproductive glands also stir up the oil production in your skin. It's the extra oil that causes acne. If one or both of your parents had acne when they were young, then the odds are increased that you will too.

If you have just a few pimples on your face every now and then, I can assure you that you notice them much more than anyone else does. I've been self-conscious enough about a pimple on my nose or forehead to ask a friend, "So how bad does my pimple look?" The response has always been the same, "What pimple?" Think about your friends, do you know how many pimples are on their faces?

Developing acne before you get your period can be a sign that a more serious case is on the way. If you have to contend with a lot of pimples on a regular basis, first know that you have my sympathy—acne sucks. Take some comfort in the fact that once puberty settles down, your acne will likely disappear. Take even more comfort in the fact that there's been a lot of recent medical advancement in treating acne. The action tips will have you covered.

> Eating chocolate and pizza or thinking about sex will not make you break out.

**Oily Hair** is another result of that annoying increased oil production. Some girls develop the greasies, while others still have to contend with the dry frizzies. Either way, there's hope. Not because the labels on shampoos and conditioners say for oily, dry, or normal hair (there's actually very little difference between these products), but because there are tips to follow.

While your hair has a natural tendency toward oily or dry, a lot of what you might do to style it will throw it even more off balance. For example, mousse will make oily hair greasier, and blow-drying will damage all hair types and dry out dry hair even more. While all through my youth I blow-dried my hair, I am now a big fan of the natural look. In college I made an amazing discovery; I met a woman whose hair was curly and full of body and asked her what she did to it. Her answer was, "Nothing." Ever since, I've let my hair dry naturally and I love it.

If you're addicted to blow-drying your hair like I used to be or to using a styling product, experiment with a natural look and see what happens. Choose a weekend or school vacation when socializing is at a lull to give it a try. Buy hair accessories and play with different styles of ponytails and barrettes.

To keep you hair healthy and beautiful, get it cut on a regular basis, periodically change your brand of shampoo, and follow these tips depending upon your hair type.

### ACTION: Managing the Greasies
**1. Cutting Down on Pimple Production.**
**a. Don'ts:**
- If pimples start popping up, don't pop back. That will only lead to infection and even potential scarring for life. If you have to pop something, buy some bubble wrap.
- Trying to tan your pimples into oblivion is also a no-no. It will only make your skin worse. Besides, the sun can give you moles that may develop into skin cancer! (Always use a sunscreen with an SPF of at least 15. An SPF of 30 is even better.)
- Putting some type of cover-up on a few pimples will often call more attention to them than if you just let them be.
- Here's a simple tip I bet you didn't know: Avoid touching your face because your hands can add oil and dirt.

**b. Do's:**
- Drink lots of water and eat healthily.
- Wash your face regularly with warm water and mild soap, and avoid hard scrubbing.
- If you have a serious acne problem, consult your doctor. There are many medications these days that can help. Researchers have been busy developing a lot of new creams and lotions that are effective with few side effects.

**2. Haircare for Oily Hair.**
**a. Don'ts:**
- Over-conditioning your hair adds to the oils; use conditioner every *other* time you shower.
- Hair styling products like gels and mousses add more greasies.

**b. Do's:**
- Consider washing your hair every day with a mild or regular shampoo.

- Try a hairstyle that keeps your hair off your face because oily skin and oily hair swap grease.

**3. Haircare for Dry Hair.**

**a. Don'ts:**

- Watch out for hair products that contain alcohol—major drying effect.
- As you might imagine just from the word "drying" in blow-drying, extra heat to your hair is dry frizzies waiting to happen. If you do blow-dry, then towel-dry your hair first to remove excess moisture. When you dry it, use the lower heat settings, keep the dryer several inches away from your scalp, and keep it moving. Once you've got your hair behaving as you want, let it dry on its own for the rest of the time.

**b. Do's:**

- Wash it every other day with a mild or conditioning shampoo.
- Make sure to rinse well because shampoo residue causes dryness.
- Condition every time you wash; it will give your hair nutrients, moisturizer, and, depending on the brand, possibly even protection from the sun.

---

Did anyone ever tell you that brushing your hair 100 times would make it shine? The misguided thinking behind this advice is that brushing would stimulate the oils in your scalp. The truth is, very little oil would be released, and if it were, your hair would become greasy, not glistening. For shine, simply keep your hair clean and healthy.

---

## Body Shape

**Thighs** and **hips** typically get larger during the mid to later years of puberty because your body deposits fat in those areas. "Why does it have to be there?" you might moan.

"Why can't it all go to my breasts?" The breasts supply the milk for a baby once it's born, but what is the fetus going to eat in the womb? It eats some of what the mother eats, but if the mother isn't taking in enough nutrients, then the fetus will pull from the mother's fat reserves. So if you choose to have a baby someday, your thighs and hips will help to make sure that the baby is a healthy one. After nine months of growing in the womb, the baby will need to get out; puberty helps you prepare for this possibility by widening your hips.

> Before puberty hits, the fat on girls' and boys' bodies is distributed in a similar fashion. With puberty, boys actually lose fat from their buttocks and thighs, while girls gain fat in that very same area—their thighs and hips.

**Height** increases throughout puberty, usually stopping approximately one to three years after you get your period. Have you heard of the famous "growth spurt"? It really does come and go in a flash; for a period lasting less than a year, you'll grow maybe four inches instead of two. If you shoot up tall at a young age, people you meet may assume you're older than you are. If you stay petite like I did, people will probably underestimate your age. If you feel pressure to act older or younger than you really are, just slip into the conversation what grade you're in or what you did for your _____ (fill in the blank) birthday.

> Do you know why a rapid increase in shoe size often marks the beginning of the growth spurt? It's because feet, arms, and legs grow faster than the backbone.

**Weight** will likely increase during puberty because you are developing and growing, but as you grow taller, pudginess from your younger years could actually disappear. It is as if you're being stretched upwards.

Your body has a preprogrammed course it's determined to follow, meaning that your genes have a big say in what size jeans you wear. Every one of us, you, me, your mom, has a **set point** weight, just like we have predetermined eye and hair color. Your body may fluctuate around the set point number by a few pounds, but basically it knows where it wants to be. The weight that your body wants to settle into is generally a healthy one; remember, your genes are rooting for you to survive and thrive.

> A generation ago, the typical model weighed eight pounds less than the average woman. Now, the average model weighs much less—*23* percent less.

### ACTION: Going with Your Body's Flow

1. **Your Curves.** When hips and thighs appear, consider it initiation into the sisterhood and enjoy your curves. A benefit I found for myself is that the additions to the lower part of my body gave me more balance and stability.
2. **Stand Up, Stand Straight.** I'm sounding like your grandmother again, aren't I? But the truth is that your body is beautiful and you should be proud to walk through life with your head held high.
a. **If you're especially tall**, you may be tempted to slouch to fit in with everybody else. Let them look up to you. We were made to be different heights.
b. **If you're short**, you may feel like you just disappear anyway, so why not slouch? You're wrong; people will notice you no matter how tall or short you are, it's how you carry yourself that counts.
3. **Don't Mess with Your Weight.** So many girls who are at a healthy normal weight consider themselves

to be overweight. So if you're considering dieting—don't do it. Instead, make sure to read the chapter on living the trim lifestyle. If you're concerned that your weight is too low, then definitely consult a doctor.

## Putting It All Together

So you've got a grasp on all the individual changes, but you want a better sense of how they actually occur. Everybody's story is different; here's mine, reporter-style:

- Age 9: I developed an odd delusion that I couldn't reach the age of 10 without having achieved a certain height. Needless to say, I stayed short and turned ten.
- Age 10: Summer camp, I'm taking an outdoor shower in back of the bunk and a girl starts pointing to my vagina. I look down and lo and behold, there they are—the first sprouts of pubic hair. (That was the last time I showered in front of others.)
- Age 10: School, rumor going around that I'm wearing a bra. False alarm—undershirt mistaken for a bra.
- Age 11: I greet my breast buds with an "I'm glad to see you," and my period arrives.
- Ages 12–13: I mentally encourage my breasts to grow— "Come on, girls, keep going, keep going"—but they seem to be content where they are.
- Age 14: My figure is so slender that I have to shop for size 0 jeans at a store called the Minishop.
- Somewhere between ages 15 and 18, I stop growing taller.
- Age 18: My hips finally blossom and puberty completes itself.

### ACTION: Charting the Course

It might be fun to keep track of all the developments that will be happening to your body. If you have a daughter years from now, you could show her the chart and let her know what her genes might have in store for her. Add a story to keep the memory alive, even if it is an embarrassing one. Someday you might even laugh when you read it.

| DEVELOPMENT | AGE | STORY |
|---|---|---|
| *Breast buds blossoming* | | |
| *Nipples enlarging* | | |
| *Areola appearing* | | |
| *Breasts growing* | | |
| *Pubic hair surfacing* | | |
| *Menstrual bleeding begins* | | |
| *Underarm hair sprouting* | | |
| *B.O. emanating* | | |
| *Leg hair growing* | | |
| *Pimples popping up* | | |
| *Thighs thickening* | | |
| *Hips widening* | | |

## Growing Upwards and Outwards: How Fast and How Far?

In junior high school, everybody was developing into very different shapes from each other. Fortunately, nobody around me was attaining the perfect "beauty ideal" of being tall, thin, and big-breasted, so I didn't feel left out. My ballet pals were skinny, tall, and small-chested, while other friends were generally medium height, some slender and some plump. This isn't surprising, considering that the beauty ideal is possible for fewer than five percent of all girls. When I think of this ideal, I like to think of a tall file cabinet with the second drawer from the top being full and open, while the rest of the drawers are light and tucked in. What would happen? The cabinet would fall over. Now imagine Barbie. Isn't it amazing that she can even stand?

To look like Barbie, you'd have to be 5'7", weigh 100 pounds and have several ribs removed. A young woman had more than 20 plastic surgeries in an effort to reach Barbie's proportions—and still couldn't match them.

I was pleased with my perky breasts until age 16 when I visited an older friend at her college orientation program and heard a guy make some lewd comment about wanting a woman with big breasts. It just took one comment to sell me on the notion that once I got to college I wouldn't have boyfriends anymore because I was small-chested. Well, what do you think happened to me at college? I learned just how silly my thought was; I was more popular than I had been in high school. I read a survey once that said that 50 percent of men had no preference for chest size one way or the other; 25 percent preferred big; and 25 percent preferred small. We're all winners.

What guys seem to like shouldn't be the basis for how we females feel about our bodies anyway. This gives guys way too much power over us and means that we put our self-confidence in the hands of fickle boys who don't really know yet what they prefer. Boys talk *as if* they know exactly what they like because that's how they think they're supposed to behave. Each boy has crushes on a variety of girls, and each looks different from the others. I know that who I had crushes on kept changing—how about you?

While I was feeling insecure about my small breasts, some girls who had developed early were also feeling self-conscious about their large breasts. They were unhappy with the attention and comments sent their way. Boys talk about big breasts all the time because our culture tells them that's what manly boys do. Do we think about their penis size? How would they like it if we yelled out as they passed by, "Boy, you're really packing a whopper in those pants"?

Sometimes large-chested girls find that people jump to certain conclusions about their personalities based on chest size. A common misguided assumption is that the girls are sexually active just because they're developed. If this happens to you, the important thing is to continue being yourself and not let people's crazy notions alter that. Stick with friends who really want to get to know *you*.

If your breasts grow especially large, you may find that your back aches and that it's difficult to stand up straight. There's help. The first step would be to go to a department store and ask a saleslady for a bra that gives you a lot of extra support. If you're still in pain when puberty has completed its development course, you could consult a doctor on whether or not breast reduction surgery would help.

## What's She Got That I Don't?

So other girls are developing at different paces from you and you can't help but notice. When you meet another girl for the first time, is the first thing you focus on her appearance and how it compares to yours? Do you wind up wanting something that she has? If so, know that it's very human to want what somebody else has that you don't. We could start a new phrase: "Well, that's just *so human*."

My favorite grass-is-always-greener story comes from when I was traveling in Africa with a woman who could have been the stand-in look-alike for the actress Sigourney Weaver. I secretly envied her large chest, while she openly expressed her jealousy of my slender form. Both of us wanted to be the other—what irony. If we *had* been able to do the old body switcheroo for a day, we probably would have gone to bed praying to wake up as ourselves again. That story line could make a fun short story; if you write it, please send me a copy through my website.

In the 1800s, teen girls weren't worried about their weight or breast size; they wished for small hands and feet. Large feet and hands suggested a rough, working-class way of life. Even the Princess Victoria, who became Queen of England, was concerned that her hands were too large.

### ACTION: Avoiding Comparing Yourself to Others

1. **Go Beyond Body:** When you're in the company of a girl and find yourself sizing up your body to hers, ask yourself these questions: Is she expressing an interest in getting to know you? What types of books and music do you think she likes? What personality traits do you both have in common? Is this somebody with friend potential?

2. **Weigh the Pros and Cons:** If you find yourself focusing on a particular body part comparison, remind yourself that every body type has pros and cons. Take being short versus being tall, for example. One evening at the movies, an extremely tall woman took the seat in front of me and I couldn't see the screen at all. She kindly switched seats with me, and then what do you think happened? The new person behind her started complaining that his view was now blocked. She confided in me that she has to deal with this all the time. Being short, I can't see; being tall, she feels guilty and gets badgered all the time.

3. **You're a Snowflake:** Always remind yourself that your body shape is like the contours of a snowflake— a once-in-forever unique masterpiece.

## Boys Change and Worry Too

In many parts of the world, girls who start menstruating are celebrated with rituals and festivals, while in America, girls going through puberty can have an especially difficult time because many of the body changes go against what our culture currently advertises as the hairless, fatless ideal. Boys, however, generally welcome puberty because it could bring what's on their wish list: more muscles, more height, more body and facial hair, broader shoulders and a deeper voice—all the attributes our culture associates with being "masculine." Of course, boys who don't attain the desired changes may feel bad. According to recent surveys, it's becoming harder and harder for guys who don't match the macho hard-body ideal. Girls and boys could join forces to get the media to provide more realistic role models.

Boys also experience changes at puberty. Like you, they grow pubic hair, body hair, and get acne and B.O. (the acne and B.O. seems only fair—that's one version of equality of the sexes). Think of a group of eleven- or twelve-year-olds that you know; are the girls generally taller than the boys? That's because guys start their big growth spurt about two years after girls, but then they quickly catch up and surpass the girls. Here's a trivia question you can ask your friends: In what way do boys develop that's similar to girls' development but you wouldn't expect? Answer: Boys experience some breast development; their nipples become larger and they get areola rings around the area. Some boys' breasts even swell at times during puberty and then settle down—no bras for boys. By the way, a boy's genitalia (penis and testicles) also mature.

Studies have found that girls' and women's magazines contain a much larger percentage of articles and advertisements on appearance and weight loss than magazines geared toward males. Men's magazines focus on activities, while those for boys highlight personal achievement and risk-taking.

# The Scoop on What Happens Inside Your Body: Your Period

So we've talked about all the changes to your body that you can see with your own eyes. These outer transformations result from all the changes going on inside your body—the changes that lead to you getting your period. It's all that baby-making equipment inside of you that's getting stirred up. You were born with all the female parts you need, but they don't get into working gear until you reach puberty. Here's what happens . . .

## The Journey of the Egg

Inside your abdominal area, between your belly button and vagina, you have all the body parts necessary to create and carry a baby. Your **eggs**, the seeds of life, are stored in your **ovaries** until they've matured. When you were born, you had approximately 2 million premature eggs inside your ovaries. By puberty, only between 300,000 and 500,000 will have survived, and only 400 to 500 will ripen into mature eggs over your lifetime.

As you approach puberty, your body releases special **hormones** that rev up your ovaries to do their job: the maturing of one of your eggs every month (the word hormone is Greek in origin and means "to set in motion"). When an egg matures, it travels down one of the **fallopian tubes** toward the **uterus**, where the egg will grow into a baby if it has joined with a male's **sperm**. How does the sperm get there? When a man's **penis** enters a woman's vagina during sexual intercourse, the penis releases millions of microscopic sperm that race each other through the vagina's moist, warm passageway, and through the **cervix,** the opening that is the doorway to the uterus. They compete against each other for the grand prize: being the one who reaches the egg first and **fertilizes** it. If there's no sperm to greet the egg, the egg continues along unfertilized. See Figure 2.1.

In anticipation of the possible arrival of a fertilized egg, the lining inside the uterus fills with blood. The bloody tissue serves as a cushion and as nourishment for the fertilized egg, which would take up a nine-month residence in the one-room uterus, otherwise known as the **womb**. The fertilized egg grows into a **fetus** that develops into a baby. If the egg arrives unfertilized, it disintegrates, making the uterine lining unnecessary so it is flushed out of your body in a trickle. This is your period (otherwise known as menstruation, which is pronounced "men-stru-ay-shun" and is derived from the Latin word *menses*—meaning month). If you see small clumps in your period, don't panic; these are simply pieces of the shed uterine lining.

---

In a girl, the uterus is the size of a walnut. But during pregnancy, the uterus expands to 500 times its regular size.

---

The menstruation process occurs once a month. The actual time period is somewhere between 26 and 33 days; the average cycle lasts 28 days. To get a rough estimate of what's going on inside of your body when, start with the first day your flow begins, then count ahead approximately 14 days; that is when the next mature egg will probably be released into the fallopian tube to begin its journey.

## How Old Will You Be When You Get It?

Girls growing up in the United States typically get their first period between the ages of 9 and 17 years old, with the average age being 12. The wide range means that there

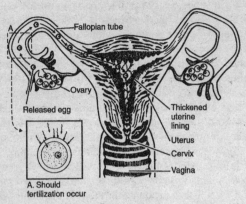

*Figure 2.1*

is no right time or best time. If you get your period on the early or late side, you might feel out of place, but take some comfort in the fact that you are in the normal range.

So if you haven't gotten your period yet, you must be wondering, "When will my time come?" There's no way to know for sure. The appearance of body hair and budding breasts, as well as a clear or white fluid appearing in your underwear, may signal that your period is due to arrive in several months, or it could take even a year or two. There's only one person who holds the possible clue as to when: your mom. The age your mom was when she got her period is the best way to predict when you'll get yours. But there's no guarantee—nature can be mysterious. Once you get your period you'll have it until you reach **menopause** at around the age of 50.

Two hundred years ago, the average age when girls first got their period was 16. Why was the average age older than it is now? Some researchers believe that it's because girls today have much better nutrition than girls did back then; since menstruation signifies the ability to get pregnant, healthy bodies are needed to nourish a growing baby. Why are girls who live in developing, poor countries today also likely to get their periods at an older age than you? For the same reason: poor nutrition. This doesn't mean that if you and your friend have different eating habits, you will get your periods at different times. But, it does mean that if a girl completely starves her body, to the point of risking death, then she won't menstruate. Also, many professional young athletes and dancers start late; due to their years of rigorous physical training, they lack the proper amount of body fat needed to trigger menstruation.

Since your mom holds your main clue as to when you will possibly get yours, do you know when your mom got her first period and how it happened? Why not ask her? Even if you have your period already, it could be fun to learn more about your Mom.

### ACTION: Talking With Mom About When She Got Her Period

Even if you feel like you don't have much in common with your mom in terms of personality and looks, one thing for certain that you do share is being female and the menstruation bond. Some girls may not feel comfortable asking, but I bet if you try, you'll learn a lot and feel closer to your mom. And when that meaningful day arrives, you'll already feel comfortable talking to her about it. If you don't have a mother figure around, or if she's not one to talk about such things, ask an older sister, cousin, friend, or aunt. Make up your own questions, but here are a few suggestions to get you started:

1. How old was she when she got her period?
2. How did it happen—what's the story? Get the scoop, details and all.
3. Did she tell anyone? Who?
4. How did she feel? Excited? Nervous? Embarrassed?

5. Had anybody told her what to expect? Or did it take her totally by surprise?

---

> While a girl or woman is menstruating, the sensitivity of her middle finger is reduced.

---

## The First Time

A friend of mine, who was a dancer in high school, didn't get her period while everyone else did. She waited and waited and worried and worried. She thought that by the time her period came, it would gush out of her like a flood, so she began checking her chair after getting up to make sure that she didn't leave a puddle behind. I'm happy to report that she got her period at age 17 and left no traces.

A lot of girls worry about how the flow will go the first time. It will catch you off your guard; that's part of the initiation process. But most girls are spared any embarrassment because nobody can tell on the outside. The beginning is often more like a trickle than a gush. If you get your first period in the middle of the night, just wash out any spots on the sheets with cold water and soap. We all have a story to tell about the first time we get "it." You will too. Here's my rather uneventful initiation:

> I was home alone on a weekend afternoon doing homework, and getting my period was the last thing on my mind. Besides, only one girl in my class had gotten hers already; the topic wasn't much on anybody's mind. I noticed that my stomach, or I thought it was my stomach, felt a little strange. Thinking that I had to go to the bathroom, I went, only to find that my underwear had dark, crusty, rusty red stains. I panicked, thinking something was terribly wrong with

*me. "Was it something I ate? Some terrible disease?" Once I realized what it was, another panic hit, "Would I have to use tampons and have my mother help me?" I turned bright red with embarrassment just thinking about it. Not knowing what to do, I stayed in the bathroom, until Mom came home . . .*

*Fortunately she gave me a pad, not a tampon— easy as one-two-three. Then the day was mine; Mom decided we should celebrate. It was like my birthday all over again; we ate at a restaurant, went shopping, and saw a movie of my choice. The celebration didn't end there. When I arrived at school two days later, the girls were lined up at the classroom door waiting to give me a light pat on the tush—their way of saying congratulations; the boys had no idea what was going on. My best friend had told the girls, but I didn't mind; it was kind of fun to be the center of attention for those five minutes. My celebrity status soon faded and it was school day as usual . . .*

I enjoyed the fact that everybody helped me mark the occasion, even if I didn't particularly enjoy the slaps on my butt. I was lucky that the people in my life responded with celebration. Here are a few thoughts on how you can mark the occasion of your first period. (If you've already had your first period and felt alone in the experience, then also go on to tips 3–5.)

### ACTION: Celebration

1. **Feel Proud.** You are joining the sisterhood.
2. **Share the News.** Tell the people to whom you feel close; let them know you've been initiated into the sisterhood. If they don't respond with the enthusiasm you hoped for, don't let them spoil your special moment. Go on to the other three remaining tips.

3. **Write Your Story in a Journal.** Make sure to include how you were feeling and what you were thinking each step of the way.
4. **Send Me Your Story.** Visit my Website *The-GirlsGuides.com* and let me know how it was for you.
5. **Back to Normal.** After that first day or two, it's generally life as usual. People will be treating you just as they always did. While your body may be racing ahead in terms of womanly maturity, it's perfectly normal for you to think and feel just how you did before the big day.

---

Women have won Olympic medals while having their periods. Exercise can even lessen menstrual cramps.

---

## How Does the Flow Go?

How does the flow feel? Most of the time the menstrual blood is trickling out so slowly that you can't even feel it. Sometimes you can detect a little seepage, like a tiny squirt of liquid escaping, especially when you change positions (e.g., stand up). When you urinate, the fluid turns the toilet bowl water reddish-pink and you'll leave your mark on the toilet paper as well.

Usually during the first year or so, the flow is extra light and might skip a month or two, or even six, or come on an unpredicted date. Don't be worried—this is normal. The heaviness of the flow will vary from month to month and from girl to girl. Once your period becomes regular, the discharge often starts with a steady flow and then trickles off, lasting a total of three to five days, maybe even up to seven. There's no reason why you can't be just as active as you always are. Jump into the swimming pool—anything goes, just as long as you're wearing a tampon when you're in the water.

In the late 1800s, a prominent medical professor used menstruation as an excuse to strongly recommend that women not be allowed to attend college. He insisted that academic challenge used too much brainpower, drawing energy away from the ovaries and causing physical and emotional damage. Instead, he said women should learn housekeeping skills because they encourage regular periods. We've come a long way, baby!

## Pads, Panty Liners, Tampons. What's the Difference?

All types of protection absorb the blood flow. A **pad** is like a thin soft sponge with a gauzy covering and a sticky strip on the underside. You just peel off the paper strip covering the adhesive and stick it right onto your underwear. Pads are easy, so they're usually the first form of protection girls use. **Panty liners** are like pads, only thinner, and are used when your flow is light or as a protection when you're expecting your period.

A **tampon** is a small, compact bundle of cotton fibers with a string as a tail on one end. Tampons come in all different sizes to accommodate light to heavy flows. The tampon is inserted into the vagina to absorb the flow of blood, and the string hangs down as a way for you to pull the tampon out when it's time to change it. For most brands, the tampon comes inside of a cardboard tube (an applicator) that helps you guide the tampon into your vagina; then it glides right out and is thrown away. The whole process is painless. The package includes a diagram with detailed instructions, but it never hurts to have some in-person guidance from a mom, sister, or friend.

Ever heard the myth that after a girl uses a tampon, she's
no longer a virgin? Well, never fear, it's just a myth. Being
a virgin refers only to not having had sexual intercourse
with a male.

My first try at tampon insertion was a scene out of television comedy. A friend coached me and cheered me on as
I attempted to insert a tampon, but the more attempts I
made, the less far in it would go. I was convinced that
something was wrong with my body; I was a mutant—my
vagina looked like a vagina on the outside, but really it led
nowhere. As you've probably guessed, I was so nervous
that my vaginal muscles were tensing up, preventing the
tampon from entering. Needless to say, I gave up. A year
later I was more relaxed and happily using tampons. A little
practice always helps, but wait until you get your period to
try inserting a tampon; otherwise, eek! Your vagina is too
dry and it won't go anywhere.

How do you know when to change your pad or tampon?
With a pad it's easy to see—it's really red. Just wrap the
pad in toilet paper and throw it in the garbage (if you throw
it in the toilet, it will probably clog the pipes—time to call
the plumber). With a tampon, it's good to wear a panty
liner as well, and then you can see when the blood runneth
over. If you lose sight of the string, don't worry, the tampon
can't sneak off anywhere—your cervix holds it in place.
It's important to change your tampons at least every four
to six hours because there's a rare but serious disease called
toxic shock syndrome that can develop if you leave it in
too long. Since at night you hopefully sleep for eight to ten
hours, you can wear a pad and, if you like, add a towel on
top of the bedsheet.

### ACTION: Why Not Be Prepared?

There are so many feminine hygiene products on the drug-
store shelves that it's easy for you to find the ones you like

best. No matter what you're wearing—shorts, bathing suit, skirt, pants—you'll be able to hide the fact that you're wearing protection. To prepare for getting your period:

1. **Buy an Assortment.** You, along with a friend or your mom, could buy a variety of pads and tampons. Take them out of the box, unwrap them, take them apart and examine how they work.

2. **Pack a Pouch.** If you like, put a couple of pads and panty liners into a little zippered pouch and keep them at the bottom of your school bag.

3. **If You Find Yourself at School Without.** Don't worry; stuffing toilet paper or clean paper towels into your undies will buy you some time as you find a friend or go to the school nurse, who should always have a pad handy.

---

The first sanitary napkins were made from pieces of folded cloth. Later, pads like we have today were developed, but there was no adhesive strip, so women had to pin them to a special belt. Quite an awkward contraption!

---

## What's All This Talk about PMS?

When I was growing up, my mom often suffered from something called PMS. For years, I had no idea what this mysterious illness was, I only knew that having it put my mother in a bad mood, even made her sad. Since neither my father nor brother ever complained about it, I figured it wasn't contagious; so I wasn't too worried about catching it.

Then I started getting my period and learned firsthand what PMS was all about. During the week before my period was due, I was on an emotional roller coaster. One hour I was angry at any person who crossed my path. The next hour, I felt like bursting into tears. It was good to learn that this seemingly bizarre behavior was quite normal for a menstruating girl. Eventually I got used to it; now it's not such a big deal. Below, I'll share with you the coping tips I developed over the years.

PMS (Premenstrual Syndrome) is made up of emotional and physical symptoms that you may experience seven to ten days before your period arrives. Some girls have only a few symptoms and barely notice them, while others may have many. Once you've been menstruating for a while, you might start to recognize certain changes in how your mood and body feels. Here's a list of possible symptoms. If you already have your period, or when you get your period, check off any symptom you experience before or during your period:

> Recent research found that going on a vegan vegetarian diet (meaning that they consumed no animal products, including meat, dairy, and eggs) has the potential to significantly lessen a woman's PMS symptoms and menstrual pain.

## THE PMS CHECKLIST
### Emotional Symptoms
___ **Feeling anxious**; the smallest thing can make you nervous
___ **Feeling irritable**; everything and everybody seems to get on your nerves
___ **Feeling tired**, yet not sleeping very well
___ **Feeling sad**, and sometimes weepy, like you want to cry but don't know why
___ **Feeling restless**; having difficulty concentrating on school work and activities
___ **Feeling worthless**; your self-confidence flies out the window
### Physical Symptoms
___ **Cramps** (aches and pains) in the abdominal (stomach) area, right before and during your period
___ **Bloated stomach**; the body retains water, causing slight temporary weight increase

___ **Headaches**
___ **Upset stomach** or constipation
___ **Breast tenderness**

### *ACTION: Putting PMS in Its Place*

If you've checked a few symptoms, you know that PMS can be a drag. But you don't have to accept PMS lying down in a weepy heap. These are ways to fight back:

1. **Mind Over Matter.** My favorite weapon against the downer emotions of PMS is the mind. On a personal calendar, make a red mark through the seven-to-ten-day period before your period is due. If you start feeling sad, nervous, or irritable look at the calendar. If you're into the red period, then keep saying to yourself, "In just a few days I'll be smiling with the sun again. I won't let PMS get the better of me." Also, be good to yourself—play your favorite music, wear your favorite clothes, and read a fun book.

2. **Choose Your Foods Carefully.** Notice that I didn't include "eat your favorite foods." That's because being extra careful about what you eat helps reduce PMS. If the foods you adore fit the following criteria, then by all means, go for it; eat healthy foods, such as fresh fruits and vegetables (Chapter 6 has tips for good nutrition), and avoid sugar, red meat, salt, and caffeine.

3. **Move Your Body.** Get a lot of exercise, three to five times during the PMS week (Chapter 4 will help you find an activity you love). Exercise releases endorphins which are natural substances in your body that make you feel happy.

4. **Get a Good Night's Sleep.** Put extra effort into getting a good night's sleep. Since PMS can cause insomnia, you want to make sure you've had a good physical workout and get to bed a little earlier than usual (Chapter 4 (p. 106) has tips for getting a good night's sleep).

**5. Ask the Doc.** If you try tips one to four and find that your PMS is still bad, then ask a doctor if there are any special vitamins or medications s/he can recommend or prescribe. Cramps can also be treated with a hot water bottle.

---

Victorian girls who were menstruating would spend their days lying down with hot flatirons on top of them to soothe their cramps.

---

## The Miracle of Life

So why do females suffer through PMS symptoms and blood management with, overall, not too many complaints? Because all of this inconvenience means that someday, probably after years and years of spending money on tampons and pads, they might choose to give life by having a baby. In junior high and high school, boys are thinking about too many other things to be jealous of the fact that someday you can give birth, but I've known plenty of men who are envious of our reproductive organs. Sure, male sperm are essential to the process, but it's we females that get to feel a brand new life growing inside of us for nine months and feed the baby from our own breasts. So if you're feeling like PMS is a drag, remind yourself how cool it is to be a female.

---

Does a woman always need to have sexual intercourse with a man in order to become pregnant? Not anymore. Modern day technology has made it possible for women to become **artificially inseminated**: a process in which semen containing sperm are medically introduced into her body.

---

Going through puberty awakens your sexual feelings, which can be confusing and exciting at the same time. Plus, entering puberty also means that sex can lead to getting pregnant. So what would a girl's body book be without a chapter about kissing, feeling pleasure, and sex? Since this book is all about girlpower and being good to your body, the next chapter on sex will help you feel in charge of how sexual you want to be and when. Just turn the page....

## Check Out These Resources

### Phone Numbers and Websites

*http://www.virtualkid.com*: Ask your questions about puberty and get answers from a doctor. Click on the PUBERTY101 forums called "Ask the Doc."

General crisis counseling: Kid Save Hotline: (800) 543-7283 or The National Runaway Switchboard: (800) 621-4000.

*zaphealth.com*: This site provides information for teens on sex, drugs, alcohol, mental health, family problems, skin problems, weight issues, and sports injuries. You can ask an expert for advice.

### Books

Bolden, Tonya, ed. *33 Things Every Girl Should Know: Stories, Songs, Poems, and Smart Talk by 33 Extraordinary Women*, New York: Crown, 1998.

Emme, Daniel Paisner. *True Beauty: Positive Attitudes and Practical Tips from the World's Leading Plus-Size Model*. New York: Putnam Publishing Group, 1997.

Howarth, Enid, and Jan Tras. *The Joy of Imperfection*. Minneapolis, Minnesota: Fairview Press, 1996.

Madaras, Lynda, and Area Madaras. *The What's Happening to My Body? Book for Girls*. New York: Newmarket Press, 1987.

# THREE

## The Pleasure Zone—Crushes, Kissing, and...

I wanted to start this chapter by telling you about my first kiss, but I couldn't decide which kiss would count as the first. Was it when my "boyfriend" to whom I was "engaged" at age 5 quickly leaned over and gave me a little peck on the cheek? Or was it at summer camp at age 10 when Robert and I brushed our lips against each other's for a split second, and then were so awkward afterwards that we hardly spoke again? Or how about when my dream crush Noah and I entered a "make-out" contest, which involved pressing our lips against each other's, then gasping for breath, then pressing and gasping some more? Or at age 14 when a guy and I French-kissed (let our tongues mingle), and I later learned that my brother had been watching (how embarrassing!)? Which do you vote for as being the first?

As you can see, merely defining a first kiss isn't so simple. It would take at least a whole chapter just to discuss kissing, and at least an entire book to cover everything from crushes to relationships to being sexual and all the complicated emotions involved—what it feels like to have a crush, flirt, hug, kiss, go out with a guy, break up, and everything in-between and beyond. Dating can be very exciting, but also confusing, not to mention possibly scary at times. Hopefully, I'll write a book on the subject someday; until then, here's the abbreviated version.

Many of you reading this book probably are not yet at the point of sexual experimentation, and quite possibly not yet in the kissing zone, while some of you are. In junior high and most of high school, sex wasn't much on my mind. Oh, I liked boys a lot. I had crushes all the time, and a few boyfriends over the years. And how I loved first kisses! But being sexual wasn't something I wanted to do yet; I was happy exploring the wonders of making out and hand-holding and rolling around together on the shaggy carpet fully clothed.

Every girl has her own pace. Some have their first kiss when they're 10, some when they're 17, some in college, and some beyond that. Some girls find themselves interested in guys at an early age, while some couldn't care less about romance. The most important thing isn't how fast or slow you go, it's getting to know what you want and following that: Following your heart *and* your head. The following quiz will help you get a better sense of where you're at right now when it comes to sex and boys. If you're feeling more romantically attracted to girls than to boys, that's great; there's a section at the end of this chapter just for you.

## Quiz:
### What's on Your Mind?

1. When considering the possibility of having a boyfriend, I think:
   a. "I might like to have a boyfriend someday, but not yet."
   b. "I want one ASAP."
   c. "That's scary."

2. My girlfriends:
   a. Hardly ever engage in boy talk.
   b. Are always talking about guys.

c. Spend a lot of time hanging out with guys or trying to get their attention.

3. To me, guys are:
   a. Buddy pals or acquaintances.
   b. Friends or people to be swooned over or puzzled about.
   c. Mostly potential boyfriends.

4. Much of the time, my brain is filled with thoughts of:
   a. School, friends, family, and activities, but not really boys.
   b. Everything mentioned above plus boys.
   c. Dating and sex mostly.

5. When it comes to being physical with a guy:
   a. I don't feel any pressure to be sexual.
   b. A lot of people I know are doing it, so I feel I should too.
   c. I feel a lot of pressure to be more sexual than I want to be.

6. Reading about the basics of sex is something:
   a. That I could take or leave.
   b. I'm definitely curious about—bring on the info!
   c. I don't need to do because I know what there is to know.

7. When it comes to feeling in charge of my body—like if I'm the one who calls the shots:
   a. I definitely feel in control.
   b. I worry sometimes that I might feel out of control.
   c. I feel out of control a lot of the time.

**Scoring the Quiz:** An (a) response = 1 point; (b) response = 2 points; (c) response = 3 points. When you add up your total for the quiz, if your score falls between 7 and 10, then you're Neutral when it comes to thinking about sex; between 11 and 16, then you're Excited; and if 17 to 21, you're Worried.

**Neutral:** You're happy being a girl who has plenty on her mind—schoolwork, friends, extracurriculars, family—without the topic of boys or sex taking up too much brain space. Knowing that you have a whole lifetime to explore romance, you're in no rush. If someone gives you a hard time because you're not into boys, just tell them Dr. Janis said you will be romantic when the time feels right. Consider this chapter as FYI (for your information), and read it again in the future some time.

**Excited:** It's fun to think about what romance is all about: the thrill that comes from the thought of having a crush, having a boyfriend, and kissing. You're trying to figure out how you'd like to approach romantic relationships at this point in your life. You may also feel discouraged by a lot of crushes that go unfulfilled. This chapter will give you the scoop on why it's common to crush on guys who don't return the affection, and help you sort out your true wishes from any pressures to be sexual that you might be experiencing.

**Worried:** Boys and sex are on your mind a lot right now, and it may feel overwhelming. Sometimes fear of involvement is your mind's way of protecting you from getting too close to a guy when you're not ready. Sometimes fear is the natural consequence of having had a sexual experience in which you felt invaded. Sometimes it's simply fear of the unknown. This chapter will help you feel confident in asserting your personal limits, and let you know some details about sexual involvement that you may not be familiar with.

In the modern American marriage ceremony, the
exchanging of wedding rings symbolizes the union. For the
ceremony of the ancient Incas, the union was considered
official when the man and woman took off their sandals
and handed them to one another.

## The Endless Chain of Crushes

During my junior high and high school years, I had a lot
of crushes on different guys. Sometimes I'd like a particular
guy for a few months, sometimes only a week. Even just
catching a glimpse of the current object of my affection
would be enough to send my heart racing and my head
spinning. More often than not, the guy I liked didn't like
me back. If that sounds familiar to you, then know you're
not alone. The majority of infatuated girls find themselves
stuck in an endless chain of crushes; the boys they like
don't like them, and the boys who do like them, they don't
like. Experiencing so much unrequited infatuation can wear
down a girl's self-esteem, but it doesn't have to.

According to my "Unattainability Theory," girls often
go for guys who are unlikely to return the affection because
it feels emotionally safer than lusting after attainable boys.
Choosing to go for unattainable guys is an unconscious
process; you may consciously think they're reachable, but
way in the back rooms of your mind, you probably know
better. My freshman year of high school, I, along with at
least ten other girls, had a huge crush on Andy. The way
the girls flocked around him, you would have thought he
was a rock star. He wasn't interested in me, or in any of
the other girls for that matter. Senior year I learned that
Andy preferred boys to girls; he was gay. Is it an accident
that so many of us girls were after a guy who we sensed
would never desire us? I think not.

Do you ever feel intimidated by the thought of being in

a romantic relationship? Then having crushes on unattainable guys can be an effective way of keeping boys at a distance until you're really ready. Don't fight the endless chain of crushes. Just know that when you feel more comfortable with the notion of kissing and cuddling, you can break the chain then. And remind yourself that whenever you decide to get involved with boys, you will make sure that you still feel in control of your body.

Since having a fondness for unattainable guys can bring down the self-confidence, and dating sends your emotions and mind racing around, this is the perfect time to start writing in a journal (if you haven't already).

### ACTION: A Girl's Best Friend—Her Journal

Writing in a diary can help you make sense of confusing emotions. A faithful friend, your journal can always be by your side. It's also a terrific outlet for exploring your creative side (I know you have one—everybody does); being creative helps ground you when you're feeling lost.

1. **Get a Book:** Buy a blank or lined hardcover notebook at a stationery or art supply store.
2. **Write and Draw:** Put your feelings down in words, poems, drawings, or cartoons.
3. **Where to Begin:** If you have trouble starting your journal (even professional writers are intimidated by a notebook full of blank pages), then here are a few crush-related starters:

   - Describe the first time you felt the rush of a crush.
   - Write about the silliest things people have been known to do when under the spell of a crush.
   - If you could script the ideal encounter with the boy of your dreams, how would it go?

4. **Hide It:** Keep your private journal in a secret, safe place.

In nineteenth-century England, the words "pants" and "trousers" were considered obscene and piano legs were covered so that they wouldn't remind people of nude human legs.

## Rolling Around in the Shaggy Carpet

Toward the middle of high school, I broke the endless chain of crushes and began to have boyfriends. We had a great time talking, watching movies, dancing at parties, making out, and cuddling. I can't tell you how fantastic just rolling around with clothes on can feel, especially when you really like the guy. I didn't want to have sex yet. I was looking forward to exploring each new way of being physical one exciting step at a time. There was still a lot of cuddling, kissing, and touching to be done. Don't underestimate the power of hand-holding, and slow dancing either!

Why does kissing and cuddling with your clothes on feel so good? Puberty brings your body to life—waking up your pleasure zones. Your lips, mouth, and tongue tingle when tongues mingle. A tongue on your neck and in your ear? You betcha. That can feel nice too. Then there are your nipples that may feel good when brushed up against. Or quite possibly even your belly button or the bottom of your feet may be especially sensitive (I'm not talking about in the ticklish sort of way). Every female and every male has a unique pleasure map—some body parts are more sensitive than others.

Kissing and rolling around don't require any how-to directions, your body's pleasure zones will tell you, "Oh, do that again!" Just as your lips, mouth, and tongue knew how to eat without coaching, they'll also know how to kiss—just go with the flow. If a guy nibbles on your ear a bit too hard, simply tell him politely that that hurts a little, and that you preferred it when he kissed your neck (i.e., slip him a compliment). It's just a matter of voicing your likes and dislikes, and getting to know his.

---

While females first reach their sexual peak around age 30 and stay there for a long time, males hit their peak in their late teens or early twenties, followed by a gradual decline.

---

## A Powerful Little Button

The one thing I can tell you for certain about your body's pleasure map is that the most pleasurable zone is also the smallest—your **clitoris**. This little nub of nerve fibers and blood vessels is located at the top of the entrance to your vagina. It can be especially hard to find because it's hidden by a little protective hood. When stimulated, the clitoris sends pleasure signals to the brain. Sometimes arousal can reach a level of intense ecstatic bliss that washes over your entire body (an **orgasm** or "cuming"). See Figure 3.1.

---

What part of your body has the largest number of nerve fibers concentrated in one small area? Not your fingertip, or your lips, or your tongue. It's your clitoris: with 8,000 nerves, that's double the number found in the entire penis.

---

Though all girls who have reached puberty can feel pleasure from their bodies, some females reach orgasm more easily than others do. Many females orgasm from touching, but not from when a male's penis enters her vagina (**sexual intercourse**, or "making love"). Understanding your body and what makes it tingle is a process of exploration that occurs over many years and, for many of you, might not begin until you're older.

A great way to learn what makes your body feel good,

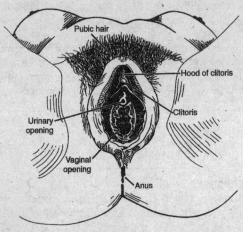

*Figure 3.1*

whether now or in the years to come, is to touch your own pleasure zones (**masturbation**). From an evolutionary point of view, we were designed to enjoy physical pleasure, otherwise women and men wouldn't pay any attention to sex; the result being that few people would reproduce, and the whole human race would die out. So when you decide to get to know your body—no guilt, please!

Masturbation is a process of self-exploration that causes no harm. All the masturbation myths are untrue; self-pleasuring does *not* make you insane, stupid, homosexual, or grow hair on your hands.

## What Do Boys Have Down There?

As a kid I was curious to see what boys had that made them different from girls. I had plenty of innocent missed opportunities. My "fiancé" at age 5 once whipped out his penis without warning to pee into a box. I was so horrified that I didn't watch. At the age of 7, in the back of the schoolyard, the kids were playing "show me yours, I'll show you mine." I wanted to peek, but I wasn't ready to show; the rule was no show, no peek.

> Ever wonder where a male spider's penis is? It's found at the end of one of his legs.

Many years later when I did see a penis up close, what amazed me most was how different the penis looks when it's soft and small (**flaccid**), versus when it's aroused, and gets longer, thicker, and firm (**erect**). Have you ever heard the terms "boner" or "hard-on" used to describe an erection? Don't be fooled by words; there are no bones in the penis and it doesn't actually get hard. It becomes firm because its blood vessels fill with blood. An erect penis grows to about six inches long (give or take an inch or two), and shrivels up quite small when it's at rest. See Figure 3.2.

> To counter a popular myth, there is no relationship between the size of a man's nose and the size of his penis. The only thing these body parts have in common is that they *both* become flushed with blood when a man is sexually aroused.

The two organs (**testicles** or "balls" or "nuts") in the pouch at the base of the penis are where the **sperm** are produced. When aroused, both the penis and the testicles are especially sensitive to touch. The sperm get swept up by **seminal fluid** that carries them through the erect penis (the liquid mix is called **semen**). Excitement causes drops of **preseminal fluid** ("pre-cum") to appear at the tip of the penis, then when a guy orgasms, semen squirts out of the tip of his penis (**ejaculation**), usually in the amount of

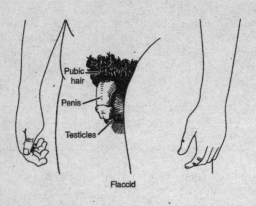

Pubic hair
Penis
Testicles

Flaccid

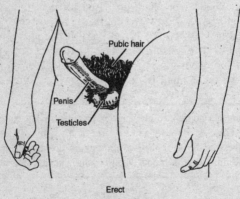

Pubic hair
Penis
Testicles

Erect

*Figure 3.2*

about one to two tablespoons. It's important to note that both semen and preseminal fluid contain sperm that could impregnate a female and that they can also carry **sexually transmitted diseases (STDs)**.

Why is it that the female organs (ovaries) that produce the eggs are located inside the body, while the male organs (testicles) that produce the sperm are on the outside? Because sperm must be produced at a temperature lower than the body's 98.6°; dangling on the outside gives the testicles a chance to cool off.

## Let's Talk about Making Love

So what happens when a female and a male get together to make love? When the couple has a long-lasting relationship based on tender caring, love, and trust, the depth of warm emotion sparked can be incredible. As a couple touches and kisses (**foreplay**), their intimacy and mutual pleasuring heightens their desire for one another. As the female becomes aroused, her clitoris becomes more sensitive and swells, and she secretes **lubricating** vaginal fluids. The man's erect penis can easily slide into the woman's warm and wet vagina. After some stimulating rubbing of the penis back and forth, excitement builds, and one or both partners might have an orgasm. When the man ejaculates, millions of microscopic sperm begin their race to see who can be the one to **fertilize** (**inseminate**) the woman's egg.

A sperm measures $1/500^{th}$ of an inch long, which means that its six-inch swim to reach a female's egg is like a human running a four-mile race at high speed.

If one of the partners is using a **condom** (or "rubber") that encases the male's penis in latex, the sperm never even enter the vagina. All of the semen are captured in the tip of the condom when the guy ejaculates. The sperms' long-distance race for the grandest prize of all turns into a one-

millimeter dash that has no reward. Don't feel too sorry for
these little guys. They live to compete, that's all. There are
zillions more. If the female is using a hormonal method of
birth control (such as **oral contraceptives**—"the pill"),
then none of the sperm can achieve their goal because the
egg is prevented from ever leaving the ovaries.

---

A popular barrier method of birth control is the diaphragm—
a small rubber cap that fits on the female's cervix,
preventing the sperm from entering the uterus. Centuries
ago, the first contraceptive diaphragms were the actual rinds
of citrus fruits (e.g., half the skin of an orange)—*not* a
reliable method. (Note: The diaphragm and accompanying
spermicidal jelly provide no protection against STDs, nor
does the pill.)

---

Making love isn't the only type of physical involvement
that brings pleasure. People touch each other's pleasure
zones, sometimes bringing each other to orgasm and sometimes not. **Oral sex** ("going down") is when people use
their mouth, lips, and tongue to arouse the clitoris and vagina or penis of their partner. This can be part of foreplay
leading up to sex or the whole sexual experience in and of
itself. **Anal sex** is when a man's erect penis enters his partner's anus (the hole in the buttocks); since there's no natural lubrication, lubricating jelly needs to be used (as well
as a latex condom to prevent the transmission of the HIV
virus that causes AIDS [see next page]).

While the only sexual act that can lead to pregnancy is
vaginal intercourse without the use of birth control, oral,
anal, and vaginal sex can all cause the transmission of
STDs, including the deadly HIV virus that causes AIDS
(Acquired Immune Deficiency Syndrome). Couples *must*
use a latex condom—the only form of STD protection currently known.

Rubber saves lives! Condoms that are made from latex rubber (not lambskin or any other material) trap the semen emitted from the penis, preventing the potential spread of STDs, including the deadly HIV (AIDS) virus. So use a condom for any type of sexual contact—vaginal intercourse, oral sex, and anal sex. Since you cannot tell if somebody has AIDS from their appearance or from what they tell you about themselves, *always* use a latex condom. But also know that you cannot contract AIDS from hugging, holding hands, or hanging out. In fact, people living with HIV or AIDS can feel very lonely—so reach out your hand.

Did any of what I said so far in this chapter make you think any differently about your body? Maybe something I said grossed you out. Just a little? If it did, I'm sure you're not alone. When I was 11, my much older cousin Nancy said that she would tell me about French kissing, but warned that I would find it disgusting. Thinking I was a sophisticated NYC girl of 11 going on 17, I assured her I wouldn't. Well, after hearing about those tongues caressing each other, I certainly was put off. But I was glad she told me. By the time I French-kissed at 14, I no longer found making out gross. One of my many criteria for determining when I was ready to try something new was when the thought of the particular act no longer weirded me out. What are some other ways to know when you're ready? Read on . . .

Everybody's tongue print is completely unique, just as no two people's fingerprints are ever alike.

## Knowing How Far You Want to Go

The question of how far to go and when can be one of the most confusing ones you'll ever face. It's not easy sorting out the pressures you feel from your true wishes, especially when emotions change so frequently. Sometimes a girl believes that people at school will think she's cooler if she has sex. Sometimes, a girl is struggling with feeling unloved and hopes that sex will bring love into her life. Other times, a girl is worried that if she doesn't have sex, her boyfriend will leave her. Sex can be incredibly wonderful. But having sex before you're ready creates many struggles, and solves none, no matter what classmates, TV, and movies may lead you to believe.

If you've already gone further sexually than you were truly comfortable with, please don't get down on yourself. You didn't do anything wrong. You just tried something before you were ready. You are still you—you haven't changed. Take a break from sexual involvement and focus on other activities, including friendships you cherish. If you find that you're tearing yourself apart over the sexual experience, talk with a counselor who can help. If you're concerned that you may be pregnant or have an STD, there are free and completely confidential clinics where you can be tested and receive medical services. The resources at the end of this chapter give you excellent leads on where to find assistance.

If you're feeling pushed toward any type of sexual involvement that you don't feel comfortable with right now, then try these actions.

### ACTION: Grounding Yourself

1. **Self-Confidence Reminder:** Re-visit the exercise on pp. 11–12 in which you got in touch with what you admire about yourself.
2. **Time Out:** Spend more time hanging out with your girlfriends and doing other things than boytalk.
3. **Reconnect:** If there are activities and people you used to adore, but left behind—reconnect.
4. **Explore Your Potential:** You have a lot to offer the world. (See the website for resources and ideas.)
5. **Read On . . .**

A gynecologist (pronounced guy-neh-col-oh-gist) is the type of doctor who specializes in helping females keep their bodies and reproductive organs in tip-top shape. The first visit should occur when a girl is *thinking* about becoming sexually active. Once a girl is having sex, she should go for regular yearly check-ups to have her birth control means evaluated and be tested for STDs (most STDs cannot be detected without a full gynecological exam).

# The Big Question

This book is about giving your body tender loving care—you are in charge and deserve the best. Sexual experiences are most wonderful when you're ready for them and in a long-term loving relationship. If you've been seriously considering becoming sexually active, you owe it to yourself to determine whether or not it's really what you want right now. Unfortunately, more often than not, a young girl who has sex winds up wishing that she had slowed everything down. So take a moment now to read this checklist; it was designed to help you assess how ready you feel for sexual intercourse, but you could also take it if you are considering any sexual activity, from kissing to touching to oral sex. Be honest with yourself—you have everything to gain.

CHECKLIST: Sorting Out the Big Question
*About Sexual Involvement*
___ I want to have sex because that's what my friends are doing.
___ I don't see what the big deal is about sex.
___ I don't know that much about the specific STDs and how I could catch each of them.
___ I don't know that much about the different forms of birth control: their efficacy and how to use them.
___ I can't say that I'm 100 percent sure that having sex is what I want to do right now in my life.

\_\_ I want to have sex because that's what the "cool"
kids are doing.

\_\_ I hope that sex will make me feel loved.

\_\_ The act of sex seems really scary.

\_\_ Sex will make me more grown-up.

*About the Guy You're Considering*

\_\_ I don't feel comfortable being completely open and
honest with him.

\_\_ I'm afraid to suggest using a condom because he
might leave me.

\_\_ If I'm feeling something that I know he doesn't want
to hear, I don't mention it.

\_\_ Having sexual intercourse is something he says he
must do.

\_\_ We haven't spent much time just fooling around get-
ting to know each other's bodies.

\_\_ He hasn't mentioned using something to protect me
from pregnancy and STDs.

\_\_ When we have a misunderstanding, it usually takes
quite a while to get over it.

\_\_ He hates condoms and doesn't want to wear one.

\_\_ We haven't been dating for more than a few months.

\_\_ If we don't have sex, I'm worried that he'll leave
me.

\_\_ He's putting some pressure on me to have sex.

\_\_ I trust him in many ways, but in some ways I don't.

\_\_ Sometimes he criticizes me.

If you checked off **even just one** of these questions, then
it seems that now is probably not the best time to follow
through on your sexual plans. You have so many years
ahead of you to have sex. Waiting until your first experiences with sex can be as comfortable and loving as possible
will help put you on a road toward a lifetime of sexual
happiness.

If you didn't check off any of the responses, then perhaps you're ready, but still possibly not. Before having sex,
take the quiz again next week and the week after and the

week after that—moods and relationships can go through a lot of changes within a short period. You need persistent feelings of tenderness and safety in the relationship. While waiting to take the quiz again, here are some essential actions to take: actions that should be taken anytime in your life that you're considering having sex.

---

What's the rush? Females don't reach their peak of experiencing sexual sensations until they're around 30 years old. Women stay at their peak for almost three decades—until they're around 60 years old.

---

### *ACTION: Doing Your Research*

**1. Get the Scoop on:**

**a. STDs:** STDs come in all different forms, from tiny warts to open sores, to symptoms you can't see at all. Different diseases are transmitted in different ways, including oral and anal sex, touching the genitals, and intercourse. Some of the most common STDs are herpes, HPV (the human papilloma virus), hepatitis B, and chlamydia. For several STDs, the symptoms can be treated, but the disease can't be cured. A few can be deadly by leading to cancer, a malfunctioning of the immune system, or other means. HIV (Human Immunodeficiency Virus), which is found in body fluids (including semen, vaginal secretions, and blood) and causes AIDS, is the most talked about, but there are others. This is serious business for people of any age; it's important to know your facts.

---

When it comes to preventing STDs, details can save your life. For instance, petroleum jelly will destroy a latex condom; there are special lubricating and spermicidal jellies made to be used with condoms. Another example is that condoms should be used before their expiration date.

b. **Birth control:** While there are different forms of birth control, only latex condoms prevent pregnancy *and* STDs. BUT condoms can break and fall off if they're used incorrectly, so a back-up form of pregnancy protection is always recommended. Learn your options and how to use each method properly; if used incorrectly, they will provide *no* protection. There's an emergency method called the "morning after" pill that a doctor can prescribe immediately after unprotected intercourse but this method takes a toll on your body and is not used as birth control. The only 100-percent-guaranteed way to prevent pregnancy is to abstain from sexual intercourse, but remember that other types of sexual involvement can lead to contracting STDs.

c. **Pregnancy:** Since having sex, even once, means that you could get pregnant, it's important to know your options if this should happen. There's aborting the pregnancy, or giving birth and either raising the child or giving her or him up for adoption. Please make note of the fact that these are not methods of birth control.

---

Pregnancy—

A girl can get pregnant at any point in her menstrual cycle, even when she's bleeding.

A girl can get pregnant even if a guy withdraws his penis before he ejaculates—preseminal fluid at work.

A girl can get pregnant the very first time she has sex—it only takes one time.

A girl can get pregnant even if she hasn't gotten her period yet—she may be ovulating for the first time and not know it.

A girl can get pregnant from having sex in **any** position—standing up, lying down, from front or behind.

d. **Making sure your partner wears a condom:** You need to plan ahead for how you're going to make sure that the guy wears a latex condom. Guys who insist on using a condom before you even mention the word are the best! Other guys may need you to bring it up. Talk about it beforehand, rather than waiting until the heat of a passionate moment when you're not thinking as clearly. Simply tell him that no matter how much you love and trust him, no matter what his sexual history is (even if he claims not to have one), you've promised yourself to use a condom. Guys experience plenty of pleasure when wearing a condom. If he won't cover his penis with latex, he needs to take a hike—I live by what I advise. Good guys are impressed by a female who is determined to take care of herself; they think, "Wow, she really respects herself. You know what, I respect her too."

2. **Resources for Your Research:** Here's where to go for all of this important information:

a. **Get a few books:** Take a trip to the bookstore or library and get a book or two that has loads of details on sex, pregnancy, and STD prevention, and also talks about the emotional component.

b. **Gather your questions:** As you read, make a list of all the questions you still have.

c. **Visit a gynecologist:** A gynecologist will answer your questions, discuss options for pregnancy and STD prevention, and prescribe birth control. If asking your mom or someone else for a doctor recommendation isn't possible, then use one of the numbers I list to locate a free, confidential clinic near you.

d. **Talk with a friend:** Is there any female in your life who you would be comfortable confiding in and who would be able to provide some smart advice? I was lucky to have my older cousin Nancy to talk to.

e. **Call a hotline:** If you still have unanswered questions or just want to talk about any worries you have, call one of the hotline numbers I list. Your call is completely anonymous and free of charge—nobody has to know you called.

---

STDs like the AIDS virus don't discriminate. People of any age, sex, ethnicity, socioeconomic background, sexual experience level, or sexual orientation contract AIDS and other STDs.

---

## Standing Your Ground

If at any point a guy is asking you to go further sexually than you want to, tell him that it's nothing personal, but you're simply not ready. A mature guy, who is genuinely capable of loving another person, will be happy that you spoke your wishes and will support how you feel 100 percent. The guy may even be relieved to hear that you want to slow down; maybe he does too but was acting on pressures he felt to be "manly."

Junior year of high school, my boyfriend had "gone all the way" with his previous girlfriend, but did everything he could to make sure that I didn't feel pressure to do the same. I loved this guy; he made me feel cherished. This is the kind of guy you want to find and hold onto.

If, however, you speak your wishes and a guy persists by pressuring you to go further, then he is truly not the guy for you. A guy who is genuinely capable of loving you deep inside his heart would never want you to do something that makes you uncomfortable. So no matter how much he says he loves you, this guy doesn't know how to love at this point in his life. If saying "No" means he walks, then take comfort in the fact that he may be a wonderful guy in some respects, but he has a lot of growing up to do. It may be one of the most difficult things you ever do, but it's also one of the most important. There will be so many more guys walking into your life over the years to come—I promise.

Why can it be so hard to stand your ground? Often girls are raised to believe that they should do whatever is in their power to make other people happy. This makes it easy for boys to push your "I aim to please" button. If you find yourself swayed by what guys say to try to get you into bed, then try this next action.

---

When somebody bothers somebody else with sexual words— sexual jokes, comments, or even compliments—this is called **sexual harassment**. If a kid is sexually harassing you, tell him to stop, and if he doesn't, enlist the help of parents and teachers. If an adult is the offender, then report the person right away to your parent or an adult whom you trust. Sexual harassment is emotionally upsetting and against the law.

---

### ACTION: Being Wise to Boy Ploys

I'll mention a potential boy ploy, and you think of your own comeback. Then I'll supply my suggestion:

**1. The guy says: "If you really loved me, you would _____ [fill in the blank sexual act]."**

You might say: _____

I might say: "For me, love means being with someone who wouldn't want me to do anything I'm uncomfortable with."

**2. The guy says: "You got me all excited, so you have to finish the job—I'll be in pain if I don't come."**

You might say: _____

I might say: "It's great that you find me attractive, but I don't want to bring you to orgasm. Why don't you masturbate to relieve yourself after I'm gone?"

Some guys will even go as far as to claim to have a lot of pain from "blue balls." The truth is that guys get aroused and then cool down all the time, maybe as often as several times a day, while sitting in class or watching TV. This gives them only a little discomfort, and certainly no physical harm; they're used to it.

**3. The guy says: "You haven't given me any good reason as to why you shouldn't [sex act] with me."** And then he proceeds to argue against any reason you offer.

You might say: _____

I might say: "My body isn't open for discussion. No means no."

The world economy is a proper subject for a debate, but not your body. Your body is yours, to have and to hold, and to cherish! Just an ounce of doubt is as good a reason as any to refrain.

**4. Practice Your Responses:**

Find the replies that feel comfortable to you. Say them out loud to yourself or role-play the situation with a friend.

---

Here's some fancy courtship action: Male bowerbirds build nests exclusively for mating and decorate them with flowers, berries, feathers, even pieces of glass or brightly colored paper. Then they paint the nest with blueberry juice. After courtship is complete, the birds abandon the nest and build a new one to rear their young.

---

## When Plans for Romance Go Awry

When I was 16 years old and my family and I were staying overnight at a small hotel in the French countryside, my fantasy of holding hands with a guy turned into a nightmare. At dinner in the hotel restaurant I noticed how cute our waiter was. So when the waiters offered to play cards with us tourists after dinner, I went along. After an hour of cards, I said, "*Bon soir*" (good night) in my bad French accent and got up to leave. Much to my surprise and delight, the cute waiter offered to give me a view of the stars from the roof. "How romantic," I thought as I accepted.

Well, the elevator never made it to the roof. He stopped on another floor, got me out into a small dark hallway, pushed me up against a wall, and started touching me. I tried to push him away, but he was much stronger than I was. I shouted, "*Pas encore! Pas encore!*" which I thought meant "No more," but apparently it really meant "*Not yet.*" My guess is that it was my language error that saved me; he probably thought I meant that I would be sexual soon, but not right that second, so he loosened his grip for a moment. And in that split second I lunged for what looked like the door in the dark, pushed it open, and ran as fast as I could until I made it to my room safely.

What made the situation even more traumatic for me is that I felt too ashamed to confide in my family. Even though the young waiter was the only guilty party, I felt somehow that I must be to blame. If a guy has ever forced you against your true wishes into doing anything sexual, including being naked or touching, then first and foremost, know that this is *his* fault, *not* your fault in any way. At **any** point during physical involvement (even if a guy's penis is already inside you), if you indicate with words or actions that you want him to stop, he is breaking the law if he doesn't. Even if you initially thought you wanted to be sexual, you may change your mind at *any* time. I keep repeating this point because it's so hard for girls to know that they didn't do anything wrong. Rape is never okay and rapists belong behind bars. Your body is your domain, only you decide who is allowed to touch it and how. Males who rape one female tend to rape many more times after that.

I wish that I had been able to talk to my parents or a counselor about the experience in France, but I never mentioned it to anyone until I was in counseling many years later. If you have ever been in a situation in which anybody, male or female, young or old, family or stranger, has been sexual with you when they shouldn't have, then I can't tell you enough how important it is to talk with an adult you trust and to seek counseling. Being sexually invaded can make the world seem like a dangerous place, but with help, you can begin to feel safe again. No matter what your attacker might have told you to scare you into not telling, you need to get yourself help by following up on the resources listed at the end of this book and reading the chapter on getting help (page 244) right away.

Even though sexual assault is *never* ever your fault, there are a few things you can do to decrease the chances of ending up in a dangerous situation. Many guys you meet will be *mensches* (that's Yiddish for "nice guys"). But since there's the chance of encountering a bad guy, it never hurts to be a little cautious.

---

**Date rape**, also known as **acquaintance rape**, is when a rape is committed by a guy that a female already knows, and probably even trusted. This is the most common type of rape. It may feel harder for the victim to seek help in these situations, but she must. Remember the female is *never* to blame in this situation. If this has happened to you, you need comfort, medical attention, and to regain a feeling of safety. Please turn to the last chapter (p. 244) and reach out for the support you need.

---

## ACTION: Playing It Safe

Attention from guys can feel very flattering, making it extra hard to play it safe. Here are some basic rules I recommend you follow.

1. **Stay in Public Places:** The best way to prevent being sexually assaulted is to not be alone in a private place with a guy until you know him very well. I learned the importance of following this rule the hard way.
2. **Avoid Alcohol and Drugs:** When you're around guys, avoid drinking and doing any drugs. When a guy knows you're drunk or high he's more likely to

see an opportunity to take advantage of you. At the same time, these mind-altering substances take away your ability to detect danger and to protect yourself.

3. **Don't Be the Last Girl to Leave:** If you're at a party, or any kind of co-ed gathering, make sure that you're not among the last girl or two to leave, and make sure that you've arranged in advance for a safe ride home.

4. **Practice Internet Safety:** If you meet a boy, or even a girl, in a chat room and are planning to get together in person, make *absolutely* sure that an adult is present for the entire first meeting. The stranger may seem kind from your correspondence, but he or she could be anybody, even an adult male who disguised himself as a kid in order to meet girls.

5. **Take a Self-Defense Class:** It never hurts to feel more confident in your ability to physically protect yourself. There are special classes for girls and women that teach techniques for defending yourself against males who are bigger and stronger. There are also many other forms of martial arts, like karate and judo, that teach self-defense and athletics all in one.

---

While in the human world, males are much more often the sexual aggressors, in the insect world the females of a couple of species can be quite ruthless. The female praying mantis bites the male's head off during mating. The female black widow spider eats her male partner after they mate; she might devour as many as 25 suitors in one day.

# Being Sexually Attracted to Girls More than Boys

I loved growing up in New York City's Greenwich Village because diversity was the norm. There was an abundance of people from other parts of the world and from other parts of the country. There were many African-Americans, Latinos, Asian-Americans, and Native Americans. Sure there were men and women who coupled with each other (**heterosexual** or "straight"), but there were also many who coupled with partners of their same sex (**homosexual**), or with both same and opposite sex partners (**bisexual** or "bi"). At my junior high school, most of the female teachers were coupled up with each other (i.e., they were **lesbian**). At my high school, many of the male teachers had male sexual partners (i.e., they were **gay**). My favorite next-door neighbors were a gay male couple.

Despite the fact that the residents of the Village were so diverse, a gay friend, Tony, who grew up nearby still found it difficult being in the minority. In high school, Tony knew he was sexually attracted to boys, but felt too uncomfortable to tell this to anybody. He did what most homosexual teens feel pressured to do: He passed himself off as straight, which included dating girls. Worrying that something was wrong with him, Tony went to see the school guidance counselor. The counselor told Tony that what he was experiencing was perfectly normal. That one meeting helped Tony get through high school and "come out" as gay in college.

If you're a girl who feels more attracted to other girls than to boys, you're not alone, even though you may feel like you are. Researchers estimate that approximately ten percent of the population of women and men prefer being sexual with people of their same sex. Sexual preference isn't just something you decide one day; you'll feel a push coming from inside you in one direction or the other. Pay attention to who makes your heart flutter and be true to that.

How will you know if you're mostly attracted to girls? When puberty awakens sexual feelings, you might start having more crushes on girls than on boys. When you start having sexual fantasies about what it might be like to kiss or touch somebody, you'll find that the objects of your dreams are more often girls. One lesbian teen described how when she was a kid, she played kissy-kissy and marriage with two Barbie dolls instead of a Barbie and a Ken. You may find that your sexuality doesn't quite match a category so clearly. Just because you absolutely adore a girlfriend of yours, are excited to hold her hand and hug her, or are curious about girls' bodies doesn't necessarily mean anything about your sexuality. The teen years should be a time of change and getting to know yourself.

---

Do you know which group of teens in the U.S. is more than three times as likely to kill themselves as other youth? Homosexual or bisexual teens. If you think you are or might be homosexual or bisexual, make sure to seek out support and find ways to celebrate your sexual orientation.

---

*ACTION: Finding Support for Your Sexual Orientation*
It's important for you to know that you're not alone. First, I list some key goals, followed by resources you can use to achieve these goals.

1. **Finding Like-Minded Girls:** It's especially difficult when most of your girlfriends have crushes on boys (while you may have a secret crush on your friends), and TV and media rarely portray homosexual relationships. Finding like-minded girls can help. This

doesn't mean that you necessarily feel ready to be sexual. You just want to have some friends who understand who you are.

2. **Celebrating Your Sexual Orientation:** Your sexuality and orientation are a wonderful part of you—use these resources to find ways to celebrate who you are. New York City and San Francisco are two cities that have a huge gay pride parade each year—wouldn't it be great to join in? I've seen both—they're like giant fun parties moving through the streets.

3. **Coming Out:** Deciding when to let your family and friends know about your sexual orientation can be agonizing: trying to evaluate how they will respond, who will likely support you and who won't. A counselor can help you determine whom it feels safe to tell and whom it doesn't.

4. **Resources:**

a. **Join an organization:** Many cities have local community groups for lesbian and gay youth where you can go and hang out. To locate the one nearest you, call your county health department or one of the numbers I list below.

b. **Read books:** The books I list are just a few that address the struggles and triumphs of homosexual youth.

c. **Hotlines:** Call one of the hotlines listed—it's completely anonymous. You don't need to have specific questions, just call to talk.

d. **Websites:** Visit a website that provides information and an opportunity to chat anonymously with like-minded youth.

## The Wondrous You

Your sexuality is a wondrous part of you, whether you're heterosexual, homosexual, bisexual, or not feeling sexual at all yet. As you develop and grow, you will be amazed to learn the pleasures your body can bring and the intimacy you can feel with a partner when the time is right. Your sexuality is yours to cherish and to share with somebody special in the years ahead when you truly feel ready. You have a whole lifetime to explore your sexuality's natural wonders.

## Check Out These Resources

### Phone Numbers and Websites

CDC National STD and AIDS Hotline
(800) 342-AIDS (800-342-2437) (24 hours, 7 days a week:
    Provides information on STDs, AIDS, and HIV, as well
    as referrals for local counseling and free, anonymous
    medical testing and assistance.)
Web site: *http://www.ashastd.org/nah/nah.html*


The Gay and Lesbian National Hotline
(888) 843-4564 (Monday through Friday, 6 P.M. to 10 P.M.;
    Saturday, noon to 5 P.M.)
Counseling and information for lesbians, gays, and bisexuals, and those struggling with sexual orientation.
E-mail: glnh.org


Planned Parenthood, Inc.
To find a clinic near you, look in the local directory or call
    (800) 829-7732 (Regular weekday hours)
or (800) 230-7526 (24-hour automated service).
Web site: *http://www.plannedparenthood.org*
They answer all questions related to sex and provide free
    comprehensive services, including birth control services,
    pregnancy tests, prenatal care, STD education and treatment, AIDS testing, and HIV counseling.

General crisis counseling: Kid Save Hotline: 1 (800) 543-7283 or National Runaway Switchboard: 1 (800) 621-4000.

*teenwire.com*: Run by Planned Parenthood, this site provides information on sex, STDs, and relationships, as well as an opportunity to ask an expert any question you have.

*zaphealth.com*: This site provides information for teens on sex, drugs, alcohol, mental health, family problems, weight issues, and sports injuries. You can ask an expert for advice.

*http://www.iwannaknow.org*: STD information for teens.

*http://www.thebody.com*: HIV/AIDS information.

## Books

Bass, Ellen, and Laura Davis. *The Courage to Heal: A Guide for Women Survivors of Sexual Abuse.* New York: Harper & Row, 1988.

Bauer, Marion Dabe. *Am I Blue.* New York: HarperCollins, 1994. (Short stories about the joys and challenges of growing up gay or lesbian or having gay or lesbian parents.)

Bell, Ruth. *Changing Bodies, Changing Lives: A Book for Teens on Sex and Relationships.* New York: Times Books, Random House, 1998.

# FOUR

## Have a Blast—Find Your Personal Sports Groove

Your body can give you the best possible present in the world—your sports groove. My groove is dancing on roller skates. Not the waltz and foxtrot, but hip-hop funk, what you see on MTV—but on wheels. Not inline skates, but the old-fashioned four-wheel kind. As funk, house, and old school music blasts from the DJ mixing booth in Central Park in the middle of New York City, my wheels whiz, my feet fly, and my body bobs. There's no other feeling like it on earth—who needs an airplane to fly when we've got music and skates?

When I dance-skate, I am truly amazed at what my body can do, swirling around to catch nuances of the DJ's beat. Whatever problems I take to the park with me, I shed with each spin and each drop of sweat. Stress? Sweat it out! As I spin, skating pals from all over the world whiz by with a smile. If the elements are right, I may slip into the zone where every twist and turn and jump is effortless. If I've really hit my groove, I bust through the zone into tingle territory—a tingling sensation that travels from my head down to my toes, electrifying my entire body—no kidding. Then when I'm done, what if I have work to do? No problem. Like a recharged battery, I have more energy than before, and more confidence: an "If I can dance on rolling wheels, I can do anything" attitude.

How would you like to:
Feel good about your body
Be healthy, graceful, and strong
Feel like you can tackle the world
Be trim and fit
Make new friends
Feel happy
Have fun!

Well, sports is your ticket. Don't just take my word for it; researchers have found that all of the qualities I just listed plus more—like getting better grades, being more creative, and raising your IQ—come along with playing sports. You can even get a natural sports high when exercise gets your body to release special chemicals called endorphins—a rush of feeling like you have no limits.

---

If you have a mild cold, don't sit around in bed; exercise can help you feel better. (If you have a fever, however, stay in bed with a good book.)

---

For my dance-craving and fast-action personality, dance-skating is divine, but for you it might be the rhythm of basketball or the flight of track or the slow fluid motion of Tai Chi that makes you feel on top of the world. I tried many different sports before discovering my groove. Then, when I was 13 years old, my mom brought me to a new local roller-rink with the introduction: "Here's what I did when I was your age." "This is going to be borrrr-ring," I thought. It was worse than boring at first; it was scary and painful. I clung to the railing for dear life as skaters whizzed by, and my butt hurt all night from falling. But I managed to push through the difficult phase (for reasons I will reveal later) into the "I can't live without it phase," which can last forever.

Sure, you've already participated in a few sports at school and at summer camp, but have you discovered your groove yet? Most professional women athletes had to try several different sports before finding the one that became their passion. Trying out sports is a lot like trying on clothes; you may have to try on several until you've found the one that fits just right. The trying-on is fun; we all have a different sports rhythm. To discover your personal sports rhythm, take the quiz on my website.

Have trouble picturing what sports are out there? No problem, just go to my website *TheGirlsGuides.com* and review the list of 101 Sports. Keep in mind that some sports are so multidimensional that they can be tailored to fit your needs. For instance, martial arts can be a high-contact sport or no-contact; bowling can be an individual or team sport; and swimming and hockey can be indoors or outdoors (we park skater die-hards shovel the snow in the winter). You can also combine different interests into one. Let's say you love ballet and swimming; did you know that you can take water ballet? With 101 sports to choose from on the website, you're bound to find at least one, if not many, that match your sports rhythm. If a sport piques your curiosity, but doesn't match your preferences, try it anyway; you may end up pushing beyond preferences and discovering new worlds.

> Cheerleading used to be the height of girls' athletic achievement. Now, females have their own sports teams and, by law, must also have their own squad of cheerleaders to spur them on to victory. Guys can be cheerleaders too.

If you have a physical disability, there is no reason why you can't participate in athletics and even make sports your life's goal. Every year disabled athletes from all over the world compete in the Paralympics. Wheelchair racing, the long jump, mono-skiing, and goalball (it's like soccer, except using hands to guide a ball that jingles) are just a few of the sports involved.

What's next? Locating hot sport spots near you.

### *ACTION: Where to Catch Your Groove*

There are so many different types of places where you can catch your groove: school, a club, community center, gym, park, sports center, studio, church, synagogue, YMCA, or YWCA.

1. **Check if your school offers the activity**; ask a gym instructor, coach, or teacher.

2. **Ask someone you know who already plays the sport**; you may end up with a personal introduction.

3. **Look into local leagues** (yes, Little League for girls!) or the Girl Scouts program (they explore nature, and do much more than sell cookies—I wonder if the Boy Scouts sell cookies too?).

4. **Take my Yellow Pages challenge**—I bet that you can get at least one solid lead on your sport within half an hour. Look up your sport's name, as well as "sports" in general. If you get a related listing, like "Polo Supplies" for "polo" (actually listed in the New York City phone book), then call them up and ask them for the polo grounds nearest you.

5. **Explore the Internet.** People who love their sport want to turn other people on to it too and a website is a great way for them to find you—a new recruit. (Even us NYC dance skaters have a site: Central Park Dance Skaters Association at *www.cpdsa.org*.)

6. **Look into special summer and winter camps** where you can focus on one activity (e.g., tennis, gymnastics, dance).

7. **Consider a nature adventure trip** that helps you push the bounds of what you dare to do, leaving you feeling like you can tackle anything that comes your way. There are organizations that lead these trips, such as Outward Bound and the National Outdoor Leadership School (NOLS).

8. **Make sure to gear up properly:** Later sections will assist you in finding the proper equipment and warm-up and cool-down routine.

---

Which sport is the only sport to have been originally invented in the United States?

Basketball. In 1891, a YMCA instructor devised the sport using two peach baskets and a soccer ball because his gym students were bored with marching and calisthenics.

---

## Busting Through the Awkward Phase

Remember all the great feelings I listed that come along with getting into your groove? Well, they will come, but it can take a little time as you push through the awkward phase. When we first learned to crawl and walk, we made mistakes and it took some effort, but we did it. Even my little cousin who would try to crawl forward, but ended up moving backward instead, can now walk forward and backward.

When I started dance skating, I had already had six years of rigorous ballet training and had even performed professionally, but I was awful at skating—anything but graceful. I held on to the railing for dear life and shuffled around the rink; a snail could have beaten me in a race. All the while I prayed that when I fell, I wouldn't break a bone. So why did I stick with it? Well, my small school's eighth grade class had a shortage of new boys to date, so I led the girls on a crusade to date the local public school guys, who just happened to skate at the rink.

Soon enough I had a boyfriend who sent me flying—not high into the clouds of love but literally flying. We would often skate as a couple, holding hands. "How sweet," you say; I don't think so. When I least expected it, he would brace himself on the railing with one hand and then swing me out into the rink with the other, and let go—I went flying, usually into a wall. Somehow I managed to survive, but our relationship didn't. What amazed me was that without holding his hand or the railing, I could actually skate. Eventually, I could move to the music and my grace came back. The boyfriend only lasted a month, but skate dancing has stayed in my life for years and years.

Skating wasn't my only awkward phase experience. In basketball, there were all those shots where the ball didn't come anywhere close to the basket, and my dribbles bounced off my own sneakers, only to go rolling out of bounds. Or how about in tennis where, if I was lucky enough to make contact with the ball, it would either go right into the net or fly totally out of the court. I could go on, but you get the idea. I stuck with sports long enough to get the basketball in the hoop and the tennis balls not only over the net and in the court, but also past my opponents. When you start a sport, you have no direction to go but toward improvement.

### ACTION: Building Your Skill

1. **Take a Class:** The best way to dive into a sport is to take a beginners class. An instructor can teach you the sport's rules and moves, as well as the appropriate warm-up stretches. Learning with other beginners means that you won't be the only person falling down or missing the ball. If you end up in a large class, march right up front to the spot directly behind the instructor. You'll be able to see the demonstration better, and if you're lucky, the teacher might even give you a few personal pointers. Don't worry about the people behind you; they'll be watching the teacher, not you.

2. **Make New Friends:** Meet other kids in the class and practice together. Who knows, these fellow athletes just might become close friends.

3. **Ask a Friend Along:** It's great to have company

when trying something new. Remember though, people learn at different paces in different sports; one of you will likely pick up the sport more quickly than the other.

4. **Pick Up Extra Pointers:** Rent a how-to video or surf the net for game rules and tips. Ask an athlete you know who has already pushed through the awkward phase for some tips.

5. **Get Out There:** Grab a basketball and go to your local court. Put on your in-line skates, helmet, wrist guards, and padding, and skate on a park path. Gather a few friends and kick a soccer ball around or throw a Frisbee. Whatever you choose to do—get out there!

6. **Keep the Faith:** If at any point you're feeling discouraged, watch the athletes whom you admire, whether on your team or in the pros. Remind yourself that these athletes started off in the bumbling phase too. Try to imagine how great it must feel to be that smooth, that skillful. Know that you too can groove, but you have to push through the awkwardness first. Recall my list of groove gains and my promise that the rewards will come.

---

No matter how much a girl lifts weights and works out, it is impossible for her body to look like a boy's body, unless she deliberately takes steroids that mimic male hormones. By the way, women who take steroids may grow facial hair or experience baldness, as well as risking strokes and heart disease.

---

## Entering the Fitness Phase

During the awkward phase, you'll have a few body aches and be out of breath at times. Be proud of your pain—you are working your body. Of course, don't overdo it and do give your body a rest in between workouts. Pretty soon, discomfort will give way to ease as new muscles get used to working and your heart becomes strong. Once you're hooked on your groove, you'll be running for the playing field, rink, or studio. But before you reach that point, it's helpful to have fitness goals. Here are a few suggestions on how to get in shape and stay in shape:

## ACTION: Becoming Fit and Strong

1. **Exercise Three to Five Days a Week for 30 Minutes or Longer:** Follow this formula and you'll be in great shape in no time. How will you know if your body is working hard enough? Sweat will tell you.

2. **Mix It Up:** When creating your fitness schedule, build in a couple of different sports. Often, the skills you learn in one sport can help improve your performance in another—sports synergy. Ballet gave me balance, grace, and strength, which helped my skate-dancing, which gave me fast fluid motion, which then helped my skiing.

3. **Build Exercise Into Your Daily Life:** If guitar lessons, a special science project, or simply all that homework get in the way of your exercising five times a week, then make sure that in between sports action, you:

a. **Cycle, walk, or jog** to wherever you need to go, and take the stairs instead of the elevator. Instead of chatting with a friend over the phone, suggest you get together and walk and talk.

b. **Running errands**, walking the dog, and cleaning your room are milder forms of exercise that won't help you break a sweat (unless your dog chases a squirrel), but can help you become fit when combined with more vigorous activities. Wash the family car or shovel the snow and you'll definitely win points with your parents (the fact that you're motivated by fitness goals can be our secret).

c. **As a study break**, turn on the stereo and dance and jump around your room.
d. **Become a stagehand for school productions**; your muscles will certainly strengthen.
4. **Pack a Frisbee or a Ball:** Heading to the beach or out for a picnic? Bring along some athletic gear.

---

Professional football and basketball players copy gymnasts by stretching before games. Go to a pro basketball game and you can see the players shoot around and then lie down and stretch on the court.

---

## Gearing Up To Groove

When I skate, I like to keep my body in good working order—I have no time to send it to the hospital for repairs. I check to make sure my skates are working well, I stretch my muscles at the beginning and end, I wear wrist guards, and I clean my dance area for teeny tiny pebbles that could topple me. When skaters ask me why I wear wrist guards since I rarely fall anymore, I answer, "They give me peace of mind, so that I can push my limits without worrying about it." My advice to you:

### ACTION: Ready, Set, Go
1. **Equip Yourself from Head to Toe:** Load up on all the equipment, appropriate footwear, and protective gear (wrist guards, helmet, knee pads, etc.) made for your sport. Make sure it all fits you well. The cost can add up quickly. Save money by renting equipment, looking through secondhand stores, or borrowing from a sister or friend. If you can afford new gear, shopping in sporting goods stores is a lot of fun; sports are so in vogue that athletic fashion is a style all its own.

2. **Warm Up/Cool Down:** Just like a butterfly has to flap its wings many times to warm them up for flight, you too have to get your muscles ready to fly. Here's the warm-up and cool-down formula:

a. **Slow start:** Begin by doing light exercise for five to ten minutes, which could be running in place, dancing to a few tunes, or riding your bike to the playing field.

b. **Stretch:** After your body heats up a bit, now do your stretching routine; stretching cold muscles is like tearing them. Perform the stretches that are appropriate for your sport—each sport involves a different set of your muscles. Once you're warm and limber, go groove.

c. **Cool down:** As you wind down, spend about five to ten minutes in slow activity mode—the cool down period.

d. **The final stretch:** To finish it off, stretch again—this will prevent muscle soreness and injury.

3. **Drink a Lot of Water:** Before, during, and after your workout, drink water, even if you're not thirsty. The body can sweat at a rate of more than a quart of water an hour when exercising in hot weather.

4. **Listen to Your Body:** If a body part hurts, stop putting weight on it for a while. If it continues to hurt, see a doctor. Injuries can be treated best if treated early.

5. **Get a Good Night's Sleep:** To be alert on the field, you need eight to ten hours every night. Why so much? Your body requires it; partly because the hormones that help you grow taller are released mostly during sleep. My favorite sleep tips are:

a. **Wear fuzzy socks:** Warm feet make you drowsy. (If you overheat during the night, toss them off.)

b. **Avoid big, loose pajamas:** They can tangle you up—you need freedom to toss and turn.

c. **Avoid caffeine, eat well, and eat enough:** Hunger pangs can wake you up—"Feed me!"

d. **Avoid bedtime TV:** If you have a TV in the bedroom, pull the cable plug—static television is less addictive. Want to see a look of shock on your parents' faces? Give them back the TV.

e. **Count anything but sheep:** Count something personal, like the number of sports you've tried, the number of birthday parties you've been to . . .

f. **Try a sleep technique I designed called The Dream Maker:** Picture a scene from your life and then turn it into a cartoon episode.

g. **Start that wonderful cycle:** Getting enough exercise helps you sleep and vice versa.

---

Many leaders in science and politics, including Albert Einstein, Thomas Edison, and John F. Kennedy, kept their energy flowing in what natural way? The power nap. If you find yourself low on energy, take a brief 20–30 minute snooze.

---

## Dress To Sweat and Be Beautiful

Some people like to say, "Women don't sweat, they perspire." Well, I'm a woman and I certainly sweat. What are other words for sweat? There's swelter, exude, secrete, drip, reek, and glow. Personally, I like glow—sweat makes you shine and show off your glistening body. Sweat is a sign of your passion. While black clothes will hide the visuals of sweat, showing off your sweat can let people know how much you're working your body.

There's the casual sporty look of untucked T-shirt and shorts, and then there's the tight-fitting athletic wear of the cotton-lycra blend. Personally, I've been converted from the loose to tight-fitting style. I used to be too self-conscious to wear clothes that clung to my body. But then, one sweltering hot day of skating, it was either shed my top layer of clothing or faint. Within no time I was enjoying the way the lycra moved with me; the loose clothing had a habit of getting in the way. Give it a try. You can always put the T-shirt back on. Being athletic is so in style that non-athletes wear lycra too.

### ACTION: The Athletic Look

1. **Shop Around and Raid Closets:** If you're shocked by the high prices of athletic wear, don't worry; there are cheaper routes to looking hip. Try discount clothing stores, as opposed to sporting goods shops. Sometimes lingerie departments have better sales on sports bras and leggings that are just like the tops and shorts in the sports department. Ask your mom and dad if they have any old T-shirts and sweats around—it can be fun to wear clothes emblazoned with their college alma maters, a personal touch.

2. **Make Sure That Your Feet Are Happy:** Comfortable shoes can still be hip. The most compliments I've ever gotten on any pair of shoes was on my super-deluxe, hip-hop aerobics, high-top sneakers. Definitely avoid hip platform sneakers—they're dangerous, like playing basketball in high heels.

3. **Tie Your Hair Back Out of Your Eyes:** Add a headband. It not only looks cool, but it also keeps the sweat from dripping down onto your face.

4. **Leave the Makeup in the Locker Room:** Exercise will flush your cheeks and lips red and put a sparkle in your eyes.

Can you imagine having to wear long, heavy skirts and corsets when bicycling, playing hockey or tennis, or hiking up mountains? Well, a century ago, this is what girls and women had to do until a designer named Amelia Bloomer invented Bloomers—billowy knickers. Females could finally shed their long skirts for sports and make a political statement of freedom from restriction while they played.

## The Stink Factor

I've definitely had sweat insecurity. When a guy I had a crush on for a while in the park finally suggested that we get together for a non-skate date, I had the following dream:

*The guy sent a letter to my house requesting where and when he'd like to get together; accompanying the letter was a bottle of perfume—a not-so-subtle hint that I stunk.*

Thank goodness that was only a dream. Reality is much sweeter. I can skate non-stop in the park for four hours, and people will actually come sniffing around rather than running away. What's my secret? It's among the action tips below.

### ACTION: Smell Sweet While You Sweat

1. **Wear Sunscreen:** This is my big secret. People love how it smells because it reminds them of the beach (and it protects your skin as well).
2. **Wear a Sleeveless Shirt:** This lets your armpits breathe.
3. **Wear Deodorant or Antiperspirant:** You can benefit from the lesson I learned the hard way: Deodorant can clump when you work out, so as a precaution, just wipe off the excess as you dress to sweat.
4. **Remember That You Are Not Alone:** Remind yourself that everybody around you is sweating too, and if not, then they're not pushing it like you are.

---

Males sweat more than females. The larger the athlete, the greater the sweat loss.

Now that you know you can sweat and still be beautiful, it's time to consider going where the action is: the soccer and lacrosse fields, the basketball and tennis courts, and more. What I'm getting at is that the best way to get a good workout is to compete in your sport of choice. Read on. . . .

## Check Out These Resources

### Phone Numbers and Websites:

Women's Sports Foundation
(800) 227-3988 (Regular business hours; Become a member and receive their wonderful newsletter about a variety of sports stars and stories from girl athletes.)
Website: *www.lifetimetv.com/WoSport*

*http://www.usoc.org*: The United States Olympic Committee can refer you locally to places where you can learn all the different sports; they're a great resource.

*www.girlsoccerworld.com*: Information for girls on where they can learn and play the sport.

*http://www.isu.org*: The International Skating Union can guide you to local opportunities.

*http://www.siforwomen.com*: This *Sports Illustrated for Women* site includes the latest issue of the magazine, as well as information on women's professional basketball, tennis, golf, and college basketball.

*zaphealth.com*: This site provides information for teens on sex, drugs, alcohol, mental health, family problems, skin problems, weight issues, and sports injuries. You can ask an expert for advice.

# Books

Blais, Madeline. *In These Girls Hope Is a Muscle*. New York: The Atlantic Monthly Press, 1995.

Kwan, Michelle, and Laura M. James. *Heart of a Champion: In Her Own Words*. New York: Scholastic Inc., 1998.

Levy, Marilyn. *Run for Your Life*. Boston: Houghton Mifflin, 1996.

Milholland, Charlotte. *The Girl Pages: A Handbook of the Best Resources for Strong, Confident, Creative Girls*. New York: Hyperion, 1999.

Morgan, Terri. *Gabrielle Reece: Volleyball's Model Athlete*. Minneapolis, Minnesota: The Lerner Publishing Group, 1999.

# FIVE

## Competition—Go For It!

There's nothing like the thrill of competing in a high-action sport—a game so fast-paced that if you stop to wipe the sweat off your face, you miss the play. Imagine this:

*You're on the basketball court and a member of the other team is dribbling toward the basket; nobody has her covered. You jump in front, stopping her dead in her tracks—she has nowhere to turn. She attempts a pass to her teammate, but you're too good for her— you intercept and take control of the ball, your teammates go wild. You dribble a few steps and then hand the ball off. You're itching to head toward the basket, but the opponent covering you is sticking close— she's your shadow. But not for long, you have her running in circles. She's dizzy now. You fake her out and make a run for the basket. You're just in time to catch the ball sent your way. The future of this point rests on you now. You dribble toward the basket at high-speed, there's no stopping you. You jump; the ball flies off your hands. Just as you shoot, an opponent lunges in and throws her hand up in a desperate attempt to foil your shot. She's too late. The ball lands smack in the middle of the basket— swoosh—it goes in without even touching the rim. Your teammates are ecstatic, throwing you quick high-fives as you all rush to the other side of the court to block your opponents, who now have the ball. The heat of the action continues—you're right in the thick of it.*

How fun did that sound? I admit that this scene wasn't quite my experience; at 5'1", intercepting passes and making baskets were never my strong points. But I still had a great time dribbling so low to the ground that none of the tall players could get near the ball, and then passing to taller girls who made the shot—the teammate spirit. Do you enjoy competition? Does competition bring out the best or worst in you? Take the quiz and find out.

### Quiz:
### How Do You Play Under Pressure?

When taking this quiz, think of a time that you played against a competitor on your own or with a team, or just imagine the scene.

1. During the warm-up period, when nobody is keeping score, you:
   a. Play better than you do during the game.
   b. Play about the same as you do during the game.
   c. Play worse than you do during the game.

2. The official game is about to begin and you feel mostly:

   a. Scared to death.
   b. Ready to let the game begin.
   c. Excited—you can't wait.

3. You're watching the ball come toward you and think:
   a. "Oh no! Why can't the ball be flying toward somebody else—I don't want to miss!"
   b. "Looks like it's coming my way."

c. "Come here, ball; I've got you right where I want you."

4. A record number of fans are watching your game today and you:
   a. Wish they would go away, and wind up playing your worst.
   b. Barely notice their existence.
   c. Love to know they're there, and play your best.

5. When you're on the winning team, you think:
   a. "We were lucky to win this one; we should quit while we're ahead."
   b. "That was fun."
   c. "Yes! We beat them and I played well; bring on the next game."

6. When you notice that the losing team is unhappy, you think:
   a. "The other team looks so upset; I wish we hadn't won."
   b. "What's the big deal? It's just a game."
   c. "I want to go over to the other team and shake their hands for a game well-played."

7. When you are on the losing team you think:
   a. "That was so embarrassing. I suck."
   b. "Oh, well. Maybe we'll win next time."
   c. "Let's have a rematch; we'll practice more and get them next time."

**Scoring the Quiz:** An (a) response = 1 point; (b) response = 2 points; and a (c) response = 3 points. When you add up your total for the quiz, if your score falls between 7 and 11, then you're Dreading Competition; between 12 and 16, then you're Indifferent to Competition; and if between 17 and 21, you're Thriving on Competition.

**Dreading Competition:** When your skills are pitted against another's, when you're part of a team that's counting on you to perform your best, when people are watching you, you perform worse than when you're playing just for fun. Instead of a rush of excitement, you feel pressure and fear, and wonder, "What if the other team will feel badly if we win?" You're not alone. A lot of girls feel this way, much more than boys do. Even if competition brings out the worst in you now, you can always turn this around. Competition can not only be cooperative, but also can give you an edge in all areas of your life, including school. Read on and I'll tell you how.

**Indifferent to Competition:** You are engaged in the sport for sheer enjoyment. Win or lose, fans or no fans, your focus is on the sport itself, and you play at the same skill level no matter what the circumstances. You can't quite understand why players around you are getting so excited when you're winning or so upset when you're losing. But as long as your team members don't insist that you become as jazzed or discouraged as they are, you're happy to let them have their feelings. It's great that you can enjoy a sport for the sport itself, but it might also be exciting for you to celebrate your wins and feel challenged by your losses. Read on . . .

**Thriving on Competition:** When there's an opponent to beat and fans are watching, your adrenaline pumps through your body and you are on! You hit your stride. You hit your moves. Pressure is on and you play your best. You can say, "Hey, world, I want to win." You may have certain situations that psych you out (like playing against a team with a fantastic track record), or special psych-ons (like if your dad's in the audience). This chapter will help you overcome your psych-outs and to hold onto your competitive spirit as you grow older.

So now you know how competition tends to affect your performance. Don't stop here; there's a lot about competition I bet you didn't know, like the fact that competition increases the intensity at which you play and thus gives you a better workout. Read on for other provocative facts that just might change how you feel about competition or reaffirm your commitment to it. Being revved up to do your best and celebrate your accomplishments can be beneficial to many areas of your life, schoolwork and social life included.

---

> Girls who play competitive sports in high school graduate at a higher rate than non-athletic students.

---

## Competition is Essentially Cooperative

Have you ever fallen into the trap of worrying that being competitive is rude? I certainly have. There's a pool (billiards) game called "cut-throat," in which three players try to sink each other's balls. The first time I played, my opponents were a male and a female. Any time the woman and I would go for each other's balls, we'd apologize; we didn't want to hurt each other's feelings or make each other jealous. We women were not enjoying ourselves, plus the guy won. The next time I played, it was with two guys; nobody apologized, the game was much more fun, and I won.

Boys are often told that they should want to win. Girls are often told that they should try their best to cooperate with others, not triumph over them. It's no wonder we've created a country in which only men run for President of the United States. Participating in team sports helps girls develop the winning spirit and enhances their sense of cooperation; that's what working with teammates is all about. As a female athlete, you can have it all.

Even your relationship with your opponent is cooperative. You're probably thinking, "Yeah, right, tell me another one." Seriously, opponents help each other test their skills by challenging each other to play the best they can. This is an invaluable service. It's not much fun to play against somebody who poses no challenge. Imagine that you're an advanced player playing against a beginner and you run the player off the court; where's the satisfaction in that? Even outshining your own teammates can give them a goal to strive toward.

> Mia Hamm, who has broken nearly every record in professional soccer and helped her women's team win the 1999 World Cup, believes that she owes her success to competition itself:
> *All my life I've been playing up, meaning I've challenged myself by competing with players older, bigger, more skillful, more experienced—in short, better than me. When I was six, my big brother Garrett ran circles around me. At ten, I joined an eleven-year-old boys' team and, eventually, led them in scoring. Seven years later, I found myself playing for the number-one college team in America after becoming the youngest player ever to suit up for the U.S. Women's National Team.*
>
> *Was I that good? No, but early on coaches detected a competitive fire in me and fed it by continually pitting me against superior opponents. Back then, I wasn't sure I fit in; after all, I was shy and a bit intimidated by players I had idolized. But each day I attempted to play up to their level and earn their respect, and I was improving faster than I had ever dreamed possible.[5]*

---

Baseball as a non-competitive sport? In the mid-1800s, the game was more of a social event. There were many intermissions in which tea was served, the batter could tell the pitcher where the ball should be thrown, and bunting was considered rude.

### ACTION: Keeping Competition Cooperative

1. **Keep Your Perspective:** As long as you don't start seeing the opponent as an evil enemy who must be stopped, then it's fine to be as competitive as you want to be. You actually have a lot more in common with your opponent than you do with most people—you both love the same sport.

2. **Shake Your Competitors' Hands at the End of a Game:** Whether you've won or lost, the handshake says, "Thanks for giving me this opportunity to see how well I could play today." Notice how I had the person say "today." Who knows what would happen if you held a rematch the next day?

3. **Be Inspired By Your Opponent:** If you lose a match, ask yourself this question about your opponent(s): "What was it about her playing that made her so darn good?" Use your answer as inspiration for your next practice session.

---

Eighty percent of the women who are key leaders in *Fortune* 500 companies (major corporations) played sports when they were young and considered themselves to be "tomboys."

---

## Positive Thinking Is Where It's At

When I played outfielder on the softball team at summer camp, I used to stand in the field and pray that the ball wouldn't come my way. You'd think that I might have been bored and wanted some action, but I just kept thinking, "I better not mess up. I better not mess up. My teammates will hate me and know how uncoordinated I am." A boy in my position would have been much more likely to think,

"Come on, ball, come to me, let me show them what I've got."

Did you know that if a girl performs poorly she's likely to think that she lacks sports ability? While if a guy performs poorly, he's more likely to think that he was having an unlucky day. If a boy hits a losing streak, he'll probably think, "I've got a lot of practicing to do." But if a girl hits a losing streak, she's more likely to think, "I make mistake after mistake. I'm such a loser," and then possibly quit the sport altogether.

---

Girl athletes drop out of sports at a rate six times greater than boys.

---

Here are encouraging words straight from the coach of a winning high school girls' basketball team from Amherst, Massachusetts:
*Don't be afraid to mess up. Basketball is a game of mistakes. Assume you're going to make some mistakes, and don't start kicking yourself until about the fifth one. My rule is that the only mistake that's going to get you off the floor is not hustling.*[6]

The saying "You get an 'A' for effort" applies to sports as well as schoolwork.

When male and female athletes perform well, boys also win in the attitude department. A guy will take credit for the skill he exhibits, while a girl is more likely to think that she was just having a lucky day. So, girls, all we have to do is think more positively. We've got to put ourselves out there and show the world what we've got! If we fall down, then we'll get back up again, practice, and do better next time.

### *ACTION: On the Road to Positive Thinking*

1. **If You Played Well:** Congratulate yourself—a mental pat on the back, "I was really good out there" or how about even, "I was fantastic!"
2. **If You Wish You Had Performed Better, Say to Yourself:**
a. **"Maybe I was just unlucky or having a bad day."** Boys allow themselves to have unlucky days; girls should too. Perhaps the sun just happened to be glaring down in your face; you'll make sure to wear your sunglasses next time.
b. **"What about those good moments?"** Think about the game in its entirety; were there any points where you really hustled, got the ball close to the goal, made a good pass or throw, foiled your opponent, or saw a strategy clearly in your head?
c. **"I think I can. I think I can."** Did you read that children's book *The Little Engine That Could*, by Watty Piper? If not, see if your local library or bookstore has it—it's quite motivational for anyone of any age. No more "No, I can't."
d. **"What was working against me?"** Are there skills you need to spend time building up? Then promise yourself you'll put in a little more practice time; ask a buddy to join you. Was your mind psyching you out because you didn't want to hurt your opponent's feelings? Or maybe you were psyched out by the thought that people were watching? Read on to learn about conquering your psych-outs.

## Let It Shine

What effect does an audience have on physical performance? Psychologists were interested in answering this question, so they trained cockroaches to run through a maze to the end, where there was a reward of roach food (which probably resembles human food, since roaches love our kitchens so much). After a roach was timed for its run, an audience of roaches was placed toward the end of the maze (I wonder how roaches cheer? Maybe they wave their antennas.), and the roach was timed again. The results? The roaches ran faster in the presence of an audience. So it seems that roaches tend to perform better in the presence of onlookers; do humans?

Human brains are obviously more complicated than roach brains. When I'm skating in the park during the summer, and there's a huge audience of tourists with video cameras surrounding our skaters' circle, I have two thoughts that interfere with my ability to skate. One is, "If I fall, will they laugh?" The other is, "If I skate well, with a smile on my face, will they think I'm a show-off?" Meanwhile, most of the good male skaters are strutting their stuff and loving it; the audience loves it too. These guys, who often push themselves to add crowd-pleasing moves to their repertoire, get better and better.

> Mia Hamm talks about how important it is to celebrate your success and continue challenging yourself:
> *Take your victories, whatever they may be, cherish them, use them, but don't settle for them. There are always new, grander challenges to confront, and a true winner will embrace each one.*
>
> *I firmly believe that success breeds success. Once you have achieved something, your confidence begins to build. You realize you're capable of doing it again. But each time you must work harder, because the old saying is true, it is more difficult to stay on top than to get there.*[7]

### ACTION: Showing Them What You've Got

1. **Remind Yourself That Fans and Family Who Are Watching Are:**
a. **Rooting for you:** They want you to do well; that's why they came.
b. **Admiring your courage:** They're thinking, "I wish I were brave enough to get out there."
2. **Strut Your Stuff:** Whenever the dance skaters form a big circle, it's always the guys who take turns showing off their moves in the center; rarely does a female venture in. I'll make you a promise; I will strut my stuff in the center of the skaters' circle next time, if you strut your stuff too in whatever you do. Keep me posted through my website.

---

Which high school sports are most popular among girls?

Basketball, followed by outdoor track and field, volleyball, and softball.

---

## Psych-Outs and Psych-Ons: We All Have Them

While reading this chapter, were there any times when you thought, "Yeah, I let that get to me when I'm playing"? Those situations are called psych-outs; your brain tells you *not* to play well, so of course, your performance suffers. On the positive side, all athletes experience certain situations that get them pumped up to play their best—these are psych-ons.

I remember a time I was bowling with a group of friends and my best performance ever turned into my worst. I was getting strike after strike and was gloriously amazed to discover that I could play that well. I was so focused on the ball, alley, and pins that I was oblivious to how I was scoring compared to my friends. Then, when somebody shouted that I was in first place, the rest of the balls I bowled that night went right into the gutter. So which psych-on of mine was in play? Knowing that I was beating my personal best made me feel like I could accomplish anything. Which psych-out came into action once the scores were called out? Knowing that I was beating others made me worried that I was making the others feel bad; as a result, my game went right into the gutter, literally.

What do I need to work on? To overcome my psych-out, I need to remember that I provide a positive challenge to my opponent, not a hurtful experience. To maximize my psych-on, I need to stay more focused on how I'm playing relative to myself than to others. Psych-ons can be enhanced and psych-outs can be conquered, but first you have to know what you're up against. What situations get you revved up and which bring you down? Being aware of your own psych-ons and psych-outs can help you build your abilities. Here's how:

### ACTION: Psych Yourself On

1. **Picture This:** Think of specific times in your life when you performed your best and other times when you performed your worst.

2. **Break It Down:** Think of what was happening that psyched you out and what got you psyched-on. Then try to figure out the principle behind why the situation affected you the way it did; in other words, what are your psychological vulnerabilities and what are your strengths? Add your conclusions to the chart below. I started you off with a couple of my own that you already know (believe me, I have more).

| *Psych-Outs* | *Principle* | *Psych-Ons* | *Principle* |
|---|---|---|---|
| Beating others | Don't want to hurt feelings | Beating my personal best | Feeling like I have no limits |
| | | | |
| | | | |
| | | | |
| | | | |
| | | | |

**3. Play Your Best:**

a. **Maximize your psych-ons.** For example, maybe working with teammates, as if you're all part of the same family, does wonders for your game; so join a team. Or you do especially well when your best friend is in the audience rooting for you—invite her along.

b. **Minimize your psych-outs.** Don't avoid psych-out situations; tackle your anxious thoughts head-on. Remind yourself of the underlying psych-out principle and argue against it. For instance, maybe you get incredibly nervous during team tryouts because your performance is being evaluated. Then tell yourself that if you don't make the team this season, you can always practice, join a community league, and then try again next season.

If a girl hasn't participated in sports by the time she is ten, then there is only a ten percent chance she'll become active by the time she is 25. Beat the statistics and show the world that girls can dare to start a sport at any age.

## Professional Women's Sports Are on the Rise

When I was growing up just a couple of decades ago, there were no professional women's teams. In order to watch amazing female athletes, I had to wait every four years for the Olympics to appear on TV. When I was 12 years old, there was a major breakthrough in women's sports. Billie Jean King was the women's tennis champion, and Bobby Riggs, a pro male player, challenged her to a match that came to be known as "The Battle of the Sexes." With the world watching, she beat him 6–4, 6–3, 6–3—not even close! Billie Jean King continued to fight for women's rights in sports.

Each sport has its own story about how a woman broke the gender barrier. In martial arts, it was Rusty Kanokogi who disguised herself as a man by binding her breasts with an ace bandage and using her unisex name. She captured the 160-pound title in the 1959 New York YMCA Judo Championships, but the tournament judge threatened to disqualify her entire team when he discovered that Rusty was a woman. In response, Rusty fought to get women's judo into the Olympics.

Female athletes had racial as well as gender barriers to break. Althea Wilson was the first African-American woman to win the Wimbledon tennis championship; her achievement was equivalent to Jackie Robinson breaking the racial barrier in baseball. Kristi Yamaguchi was the first Asian-American athlete, male or female, to win a major figure skating championship, including the Olympic Gold Medal. Nancy Lopez was the first well-known Hispanic female athlete and the first minority of either sex to gain public recognition in golf. Today, you can watch Michelle Kwan and Naomi Nari Nam in figure skating, Cynthia Cooper and Cheryl Swoopes in basketball, the Williams sisters, Serena and Venus, in tennis, and Gabrielle Reece in volleyball.

Today you can watch females perform professionally in most sports, from baseball to boxing. While you can watch your favorite athletes on television, you can also go see them up close and personal. When you're at a live event, there's always a charge in the air as the players come out onto the field. The game begins and maybe the other team scores first, so you feel disappointed. Then the next thing you know, you're jumping up out of your seat, ecstatic; your team scores! There's a lull in the action and the fans show their encouragement by creating a human wave that catches you in its force as it rushes around the stadium— hundreds of people standing up and sitting down to the same rhythm. Then you lean forward in your seat and follow the action back and forth, back and forth, until the game comes down to the final few minutes, the final few shots. You can't take your eyes off the players, off the ball, for even a split second. With the final buzzer, or the final out, you let out your breath. The game is over. Whether your team won or lost, you still had a great time. "When's the next game?" you ask, as you file out with all the fans. Go to a game and then you'll understand why as a kid, when I was asked every June what I wanted to do for my birthday, I'd say, "Yankees' game." If you asked me today, I might say the same thing.

Are you revved up to go to a game? Or at least watch one on TV? Here's what you can do:

### ACTION: Getting In on the Action

You can always turn on the TV and find a sports game or competition. You can open any newspaper and turn to the sports pages or buy a sports magazine. If you try these routes, you'll find that they all have one thing in common: many more male athletes than female. The good news is that in professional leagues, high schools, and colleges, female sports teams are becoming more and more popular among participating athletes as well as fans; you just have to know where to find them.

  1. **Women's Sports to Look Out for:**
  • The Women's National Basketball Association (WNBA) attracts boy and girl fans.
  • The U.S. Women's Soccer Team won the 1999 World Cup Championships!
  • The Women's Baseball League (WBL) of Central Florida has four teams, and the Colorado Silver Bullets is a female professional team that plays against non-major league male teams.
  • There are Women's Championships in wrestling, boxing, judo, hockey, and more.
  • Sailboats with all-female crews are entering the America's Cup racing competition.
  • The Women's World Tennis Association (WTA) is attracting more fans than ever before.
  • The Olympic and Paralympic Games come around every few years and are full of female athletes.
  2. **Where to Find Them:** These female athletes would love your support. The more fans these teams gather, the more media presence they will have. But for now,

it may take a little detective work to locate them; once you find them, you won't lose them. To start your search, use the websites and other resources listed at the end of this chapter.

3. **Pick a Favorite Athlete or Team:** Root for your favorites throughout a season. You watch the players develop their skills and share the athletes' thrills and disappointments.

4. **Read Up:** Let's say there's a spectacular athlete you adore, or an up-and-coming star you've spotted, or an underdog you're behind 100 percent. You admire her skill, her style, her attitude. You watch her play, but are dying to know more about her. You're in luck. Many female athletes today have books, websites, and maybe movies about their lives. Even if you're just curious about a particular sport, these books can be great reading (see listings).

5. **Go Local:** Watching female high school and college teams can be just as much fun as the pros, especially when it's your high school or the college that your sibling attends. Get ahold of the game schedules and root for the home teams!

---

Can you guess which two sports attract more female fans than male fans?     Figure skating and women's tennis.

---

## Never Say Never

I remember watching the figure skaters in the Olympics spinning round and round effortlessly; I was in awe, dropped jaw and all. "How did they do it?" I wondered over and over. Then I started roller-skating and tried to spin and I was even more stumped. For *six years* I wanted to spin around like the ice figure skaters, but would stop after only two revolutions. A few roller skaters could spin and spin and spin; I had no clue as to how they kept on going. I even wondered if a physics book might help me solve the mystery. Then one day, I absentmindedly spun around and didn't stop. I just kept going and going until I got so dizzy I had to either make myself stop or fall.

It's a good thing I didn't give up; I wouldn't have known what my body could do if I had. Instead of saying you'll never be able to accomplish that sport or that move, say that you can't wait until the day that you achieve your goal, even if it's a few years away. Never say never.

To stay motivated and record your accomplishments, start keeping a sports journal. For two weeks after my first glorious spin, whenever a friend would say, "Hey, what's up?" I'd reply, "I can spin." They'd say, "That's great," but I could tell they didn't quite understand. I wish I had had a sports journal then. You can start yours now.

### ACTION: Revving Up With a Sports Journal

A sports journal is the perfect place for you to:

1. **Record Your Goals and Accomplishments:** No matter how small or how big.
2. **Note Your Own Psych-Outs and Psych-Ons:** As well as the principles behind them.
3. **Write About Your Sports Experiences:** A personal account or in poetic form.
4. **Write a Visionary Story:** Imagine your rise to the top in your sport of choice.
5. **Paste in Newspaper and Magazine Article Clippings:** Keep track of your favorite teams and athletes (who knows—maybe you'll be just like that pro someday— never say never).
6. **Write Your Own Sports Articles:** When you watch a game in person or on TV, be a sports journalist.

Professional female athletes have competed against male professionals and won. Ann Trason came in first place in the Western States 100-mile race several times. In 1993, Julie Krone was the first female jockey to win the Triple Crown horse races.

## Playing With the Boys

So if we females can push our physical limits and become dazzling professionals with loyal fans, then why aren't we playing with boys? Sometimes we do play with the boys. Take school football, for example: 800 high school girls in the U.S. play on boys' football teams and this number is growing every year. Mia Hamm played on a boys' soccer team and blew them away. But why are these the exceptions, not the norm? The answer is that most boys are still bigger, faster, and stronger than girls, or at least they are after puberty hits.

Until the age of 10 or 12, girls should play sports with boys because the sexes are well-matched physically. Girls usually start their growth spurts before boys do, so tall girls even have an advantage over boys for a couple of years. But once boys reach puberty and catch up, watch out; they keep on growing taller and their muscles become stronger. Sure, we girls can lift weights, but if a guy lifts too, he has us beat. We females are designed to carry babies and give birth, while guys are equipped with the "defend the territory and protect the children"–type body. However, if you're in good shape and a guy is not, then you're the better pick for a team. When it comes to skill potential (accuracy plus coordination), boys should watch out; girls can develop their skills just as well and even have a sex advantage when it comes to the dexterity of most fine motor skills (using the hands).

Why are females able to use their hands more skillfully and precisely than males are? Because female hands have more flexible finger joints and smaller bones.

I'm sure you've noticed that even though males tend to grow to be bigger and stronger than women, their body sizes vary greatly. That's why within many male sports, such as wrestling, boxing, and rowing, there are different divisions for men of different sizes and weights. This gives male athletes an equal chance to succeed. So consider us females as being in a league of excellence of our own! But if you're too darn good and big and strong to play in a girls' league, check out playing with the boys.

By the way, the reason why those 800 girls play on the boys' football teams is that there are no girls' football teams. There's a law called Title IX that requires schools to give equal opportunity to girls and boys in athletics. So if there's no girls' team for your sport of choice, move over, boys; they have to let you try out for their team. If boys ever tease you while you're playing sports, just tell them, "You're worried that I may get so good that some day I'll beat you." The guys will laugh at this, but it's true; there's very little that's more embarrassing for a boy than to lose to a girl. Sad but true.

Don't you think that using the term "tomboy" to refer to athletic girls is outdated? We girls need a new name for an active girl that doesn't use the word "boy" and that shows how powerful, beautiful, and strong we are. Any ideas? Enter the Tomboy Contest by going to the website *TheGirlsGuides.com* and registering your idea. What could you win? The excitement that the word you invent might possibly catch on and be used by people throughout the nation. And might even appear in a dictionary someday! Or just the sheer satisfaction of knowing that you came up with a great idea.

When you compare the best performances of female athletes to those of males across all sports, males perform better by about ten percent. Females make an excellent showing considering the gender gap in size and strength.

If athletics are where your interests lie, then you can choose to carry the sport all the way by becoming an athlete or choosing from a dozen other careers within professional sports:

### ACTION: Holding Our Own

1. **Becoming a Pro:** We females no longer have to worry about whether or not we can hang with the big boys because we have our own professional leagues. If you're considering becoming a professional athlete, there are many sports from which to choose. There are programs set up year round that help train girls and boys for the pros. If you are interested in swimming, basketball, or track and field, and are between the ages of 8 and 13, did you know that you might qualify for the Junior Goodwill Games?

2. **Take Up a Sports Career Off the Playing Field:** If being on the playing field isn't your strong point, there are plenty of other options. The more women we have in all areas of sports, the more opportunities we'll create for female athletes. What careers can you think of in sports other than athlete? Here are 13 possibilities from which you could choose (let me know if I left any out):

Coach (for school, college, or professional teams)
Physical education instructor in schools
Personal or professional trainer who helps athletes get
   in shape and stay in shape
Sports doctor who prevents and treats injuries

Sports psychologist who researches how to maximize athletic potential and advise athletes

Team manager who organizes all the practices, games, and equipment

Sports photographer for print media (magazines, newspapers, books) and promotions

Media manager who promotes the team's positive image in the television and print coverage

Sports television producer who arranges for the coverage of events

Sports announcer on television or radio who provides the play-by-play commentary

Sports journalist who writes about the events for print

Sports agent who negotiates for players which team they're going to be on and how much they'll earn

Sports nutritionist who advises the athletes on what to eat

---

Girls can earn scholarships to colleges for many different sports, from basketball to bowling.

---

## Words to Exercise By

I'll end the groove section of this book with the words of a girl on a championship high school basketball team:

> *I lift weights not so I'll look strong to other people, but so I'll be strong. I take care of my body. I make sure I sleep. I sleep a lot more than my friends. I eat well . . . too much sugar, but other than that I'm fine. If I get an injury like a pull, I listen to it. I don't drink, I don't smoke. I ask enough of my body without asking it to deal with random substances.*[8]

So can you guess what the next chapter is going to be about? Yup, being good to your body. Whether you're athletic, musical, artistic, intellectual, or all of these, eating well, combined with finding your groove, will put you at the top of wherever you want to be.

---

The participation of girls in high school sports has been on the rise in the last several years. In 1971, one out of 27 girls participated. In 1996, that number rose to one out of three. The percentage of boys that participate has remained constant at one out of two. So, girls, keep on getting involved until we at least match the boys.

---

## Check Out These Resources

### Websites

*http://www.wnba.com*: The official website of the WNBA. Events and news, schedules, player statistics, plus chat rooms.

*http://www.lpga.com*: Official website of the Ladies Professional Golf Association.

*http://www.womensoccer.com*: Website for *Women's Soccer World* magazine.

*www.wtatour.com*: This is the site for the Women's Tennis Association.

*http://www.ESPN.com*: Although most of the site is dedicated to men's pro sports, it also covers women's sports and has links to women's college basketball.

*http://www.cbssportsline.com*: Includes NCAA (college) sports as well as the professionals.

*http://www.cnnsi.com*: This site includes a link called "women's sports," which brings you to the current issue of *Sports Illustrated for Women* online.

## Books

Cooper, Cynthia. *She Got Game: A Personal Odyssey*. New York: Time Warner, 1999.

Hamm, Mia. *Go for the Goal: A Champion's Guide to Winning in Soccer and Life*. New York: HarperCollins, 1999.

Lipinski, Tara, and Emily Costello. *Tara Lipinski: Triumph on Ice*. New York: Bantam Books, 1998.

Macy, Sue. *A Whole New Ball Game: The Story of the All-American Girls Professional Baseball League*. New York: Henry Holt, 1993.

Swoopes, Sheryl, Doug Keith, and Greg Brown. *Bounce Back*. Dallas, Texas: Taylor Publishing Co., 1996.

## Movie

*A League of Their Own*. Dir. Penny Marshall. Perf. Tom Hanks and Geena Davis. 1992.

# SIX

# Eating Well—Look and Feel Your Best

At school you see what your friends eat for lunch, but have you ever wondered what they eat when you're not around? Here's a day in the eating life of a real girl your age; we'll call her Lisa[9]:

| | |
|---|---|
| ***Breakfast:*** | Waffle with syrup and butter, orange juice |
| ***Lunch:*** | Sandwich with cold cuts, soda |
| ***Dinner:*** | Fried pork chops, applesauce, tater tots, ketchup, zucchini, soda |
| ***Snack:*** | A Milky Way, potato chips, a Devil Dog |

So just off the top of your head, how healthy is Lisa's diet? My guess is that you know enough about nutrition to know that there's room for a lot of improvement. To get an even better sense of how off the mark she is, compare Lisa's diet to our made-up ideal girl's diet; we'll call her Susie:

| | |
|---|---|
| ***Breakfast:*** | Bran cereal with skim milk and a sliced banana, orange juice |
| ***Lunch:*** | Turkey with lettuce and tomato sandwich on whole wheat, carrot sticks, apple juice |

**Dinner:** Spaghetti with tomato sauce, corn on the cob, peas, skim milk

**Snack:** Plum, low-fat yogurt, graham cracker cookies, pretzels

How did Lisa measure up? Not too good, huh? Now write down what you ate today; are your eating habits more like Lisa's or Susie's? Why does it matter what you eat? Eating as closely as you can to the nutrition ideal means that:

• With radiant skin, sparkling eyes and teeth, lustrous hair, and strong nails, you'll look marvelous, darling.
• With more energy and strength, you'll feel better and be at your peak athletic ability.
• With a strong immune system, you'll fight off colds and other illnesses, and spend less time sick in bed.
• With all the fuel that your body needs to develop, you'll grow to your maximum height potential.
• With more brainpower, you'll bust through schoolwork and exams.

---

Ever wondered about whether or not there's any truth behind the saying, "Starve a fever and feed a cold"? There is: Food raises your body temperature, which you don't want to happen when you already have a fever (even still, lots of liquids and some food is good). Is chicken soup really the food of choice for colds? Yes, it has actually been proven to ease cold symptoms.

---

I bet that you have a pretty good idea of what it means to eat well but that you don't always follow it. Am I right? That phrase, "Well, that's just *so human*," certainly applies here; we often don't follow the good advice our brains give us. I'm hoping that if I fill you in on how quick, easy, and yummy eating well can be, then you'll take advantage of your knowledge in no time. Don't worry—there's no talk about giving up your favorite desserts; there's no such thing as a "bad" food in this book.

## Nutrition Wisdom

So what's next? The great wisdom of The Food Guide Pyramid. You've probably heard of this triangular diagram before, and may be thinking, "Not the pyramid again." I promise you, it will be more fun this time around. I considered adding my own drawings of cows and fruit just to give you a few laughs, but I'll spare you. Here's the pyramid in its original form, your guide to daily eating (Figure 6.1):

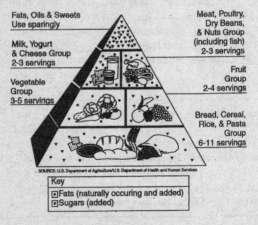

Figure 6.1

Do you know which end of the serving range you're on? It's on the higher end because you're growing. You might be thinking, "Whoa! Nine to eleven servings of the bread group!" Don't panic; the size of one serving is only half a bagel or ½ cup of pasta. Also, don't be freaked out by thinking you have to count and categorize everything you eat. I certainly don't. But I do ask myself from time to time, "Have I been eating enough fruits, vegetables, dairy, and protein lately?" and adjust what I eat accordingly. As you read through the different food groups, think about what you may not eat enough of and what you may want to eat a little less of. It's all about balance.

Why is balance so important? Because foods contain different healthful components that the body needs. Each **vitamin** and **mineral** (e.g., vitamin C or calcium) triggers a specific chemical reaction in your body that sets a particular function into action. Vitamins and minerals are to your body like spark plugs are to cars. You need them all because you can't substitute one vitamin or mineral for another, and so you need all of the food groups. Here are the specifics.

## Bread, Cereal, Rice, and Pasta Group (Carbohydrates, "Carbs" for Short)

Why so many carbs? Carbs supply the energy you need to do anything from breathing to digesting whatever you eat, bread included. What I find fascinating about these complex carbs (no kidding, fascinating) is that once we digest them using our teeth and saliva, we break the grains down into simple carbohydrates, which are really—guess what? Sugars! If you chew a cracker long enough, it will start to taste sweet; try it.

You may ask, "Then why not eat six to eleven servings of sugar instead of breads?" Excellent question! Carbohydrates break down in your body more slowly, thus supplying a steadier source of energy than sugar's quick lift-up and let-down. Complex carbs can be full of vitamins, minerals, and **fiber**, while simple sugars are usually just that—simply sugar. Fiber is to your body like a broom is to dirt because it sweeps the waste through all of your internal passageways and out of your body, clearing the deck for other nutritious food to come on in. Which carbs have the most fiber and vitamins and minerals? Choose whole grain products, like bran flake cereal or whole wheat bread, especially the kind with chunky pieces in them.

Don't be fooled by a food that tries to pass itself off as a healthy carb but is really a sugary fat. What falls into this category? My personal favorites—doughnuts and muffins, as well as cookies and cakes. Maybe if I chew my breakfast toast long enough, it will start to taste sweet like a muffin; I'll let you know if this works by posting the outcome on my website *TheGirlsGuide.com*. Why don't you try it too and let me know your results?

---

What is the main food source for half the people of the world? Rice. It's a good thing that there are 15,000 different kinds!

---

### ACTION: Pumping Up the Carbs

Any food you read about that makes you salivate, circle it for future reference. And if you've never tried one of the foods before, put a question mark next to it and check it out.

1. **Popular Healthy Carbs:** Bran flakes or a whole wheat bagel for breakfast, a sandwich on whole wheat bread for lunch, pasta or brown rice with dinner, and pretzels for a snack.

2. **Exotic Healthy Carbs:** Hot oatmeal with walnuts and raisins, multi-whole-grain bread containing sesame seeds, breadsticks as a snack, a sweet potato (yam), buckwheat instead of rice, and if you really want to impress your grocer, ask for quinoa—pronounced "keen-wa"—and see what you get.

3. **Quick and Easy Recipe:** Mini-pizza; I loved this recipe when my mom and I used to make it:

What you need:

    1 whole wheat English muffin

    2 slices of low-fat mozzarella cheese

    2 tablespoons of tomato sauce

    2 pinches of oregano or Italian herbs

What to do:

    Spread tomato sauce on both slices of English muffin.

    Sprinkle the oregano or Italian herbs.

    Place a slice of cheese on top of each slice of bread.

    Cook in a toaster oven or microwave oven until cheese is melted.

---

Did you know that the following are all fruit: tomato, avocado, eggplant, green and red pepper, zucchini, squash, and cucumber? So what's a veggie? There's broccoli, carrots, cauliflower, spinach, lettuce, potato, and more. How can you tell? Vegetables are either roots or tubers that grow in the ground, or leafy plants. When fruits grow they have a flower, and then become a fruit with seeds.

---

**Fruit and Vegetable Groups:** What's the most popular food phrase among parents? How about, "Eat your veggies." What's the big deal with veggies, or fruits for that matter? It turns out that produce is the food of life, full of the elements we most need—vitamins, minerals, and fiber—while also being low in what we need less of—fat.

All produce is good for you. The trick here is to get a variety because each type of produce has different nutrients to offer. So instead of eating an apple a day to keep the doctor away, eat an apple, an orange, a carrot, a tomato, spinach, and broccoli a day, and that should certainly keep the doctor, the school nurse, and your parents' inspection away. In other words, make sure that your plate has a rainbow of colors. Also, leave the colorful skin on; edible skin on fruits and veggies contains a ton of nutrients.

> A study found that college students who ate an apple a day *were* more likely to keep the doctor away.

For inspiration, I thought I'd include a little poem. This is what I might have written for a third grade poetry assignment:

An Ode to Fruit *by Janis*
*They're squishy, never fishy.*
*They're sweet, fun to eat.*
*Refreshing when you're hot.*
*Bland and boring they're not.*
*Packed in their own case, they travel with grace.*
*They're colorful too. I love fruit—don't you?*

Despite the glories of produce, it seems that many kids steer clear of veggies and fruit, only to grow up to be produce-loving adults. Is it a maturing of the taste buds? I think it's in the mind, not the mouth: It's no fun to be told what to eat. What you may not realize is that you've got many choices within the produce group—just within the apple category you've got more than 20 different kinds to choose from. Here are some examples from the common to the exotic:

### ACTION: Finding Veggies and Fruits That Suit

1. **Popular Healthy Produce:** In your breakfast, include orange juice, a banana, peach, apple, or grapefruit. For lunch, put lettuce, tomato, cucumber, and alfalfa sprouts on your sandwich, and throw in a peach or plum, baby carrots, or raw string beans. For dinner, have vegetarian lasagna or chili, load a heap of veggies onto your pizza, or add a side dish of salad, spinach, or squash. For a snack, any raw fruit or veggie will do, or try raisins.
2. **Exotic Fruits and Veggies:** Turn your breakfast ce-

real into a crunchy fruit salad with strawberries, blue-berries, and raspberries. Mush bananas into your pancake batter. Put asparagus in your omelet. And to drink? Try tangerine juice or a blend of different fruits—orange-strawberry-banana is my favorite. Add unusual veggies to your sandwiches: arugula, fennel, and portabella mushrooms. For dinner, how about pumpkin soup (delicious)? Discover new exotic fruits and invite your friends over for a fruit taste test; try mangos, figs, kiwis, kumquats, and pomegranates. For snacks, consider dried apples and even dried peas.

## 3. Quick and Easy Recipe: The Fruity Salad

What you need:

 ½ a head of red-leaf or green-leaf lettuce
 1 tomato, 1 cucumber, 1 box of alfalfa sprouts
 1 orange, 1 red apple
 ½ cup of chopped walnuts, or pine nuts, or sunflower seeds
 Your favorite low-fat salad dressing

What to Do:

 Rinse the lettuce, tomato, cucumber, and apple well in cold water.
 Peel the orange, separate the sections, and remove the pits.
 Cut up all the veggies and fruit into bite-size chunks.
 Put all the ingredients into a bowl and toss in your favorite low-fat dressing.

---

If a raisin is a dried-out grape, what's a prune?

A dried-out plum!

---

**Milk, Yogurt, and Cheese Group:** What's another food phrase parents say all the time? "Drink your milk." Why is milk associated with childhood more than any other food? Is it because cows are cute and go "Moo"? Or that milk can leave a funny white mustache on your upper lip? Not quite. The **calcium** in dairy products strengthens your bones and helps you grow into a beautiful young woman (did I just sound like your grandmother?). Calcium is to your body like beams are to a building: It helps you build strong bones.

If you're ever resisting milk, remind yourself that growing is a great excuse to shop for new clothes. But if you really find that milk makes you feel a little queasy or gassy, then you probably have lactose intolerance. This means that your body doesn't produce the enzymes necessary to digest dairy products. There's still hope for you; there are now pills available to help you digest dairy so you can get the calcium you need.

---

Whose milk is used more widely around the world than a cow's? The goat's. Have you ever tried goat cheese? Yummy. In other countries, the milk of camels, sheep, and other animals is also popular.

---

Are you wondering why I haven't included butter, cream cheese, and ice cream in my praise of dairy? These foods have a lot of **fat** in addition to a little calcium and other nutrients, so they belong more in the sugars/fat group. Don't get me wrong—in small doses, fat is good. In fact, you need fat in order to survive. Fat helps you grow, gives you sustained energy, enables vitamins to nourish your body, and keeps you warm on a cold day. Also, fat is to your internal organs like bubble wrap is to a fragile glass vase being shipped through the mail.

So why does fat get so much bad press? Saturated fat (mostly solids), such as that found in butter and in meat, clogs your arteries, which can lead to heart disease and other deadly illnesses. The more healthful unsaturated fats (liquids) come mainly in the form of oils.

Here are some healthy and fun ways to get all the calcium-rich dairy you need to blossom:

### *ACTION: Fun with Dairy*

1. **Popular Healthy Dairy:** Have low-fat or skim milk with your whole-grain cereal or in a glass any time of day. Smile and say, "cheese," when making a sandwich; add a slice of low-fat Swiss, Muenster, or Monterey Jack. Grab a low-fat yogurt for a snack or throw it over a bowl of fruit. Have cottage cheese with sweet peaches or cantaloupe. Make hot chocolate with low-fat milk instead of water.

2. **The More Exotic Route:** Try the "new taste" of milk; yes, they're dressing milk up now with more than just chocolate, there's banana and strawberry. Crumble feta or goat cheese onto your salad, and top your spaghetti, salad, or veggies with Parmesan cheese.

3. **Quick and Easy Recipe: Fruity Yogurt Shake**

What you need:
>    8 fresh or frozen strawberries
>    1 cup low-fat strawberry yogurt
>    ¼ cup skim milk
>    A dash of vanilla extract is optional

What to do:
>    Wash fresh strawberries and remove leaves.
>    Combine all ingredients in a blender and mix until smooth.

**Meat, Poultry, Fish, Dry Beans, Eggs, and Nuts Group:**
What do nuts and fish have in common? Yes, they both may be found swimming in salt, but that's not really what I'm getting at. These foods, along with the others in this group, have some **protein**, as well as **iron**. Protein is to your body like bricks are to a building because it helps to

build your cells. Having low iron is like trying to run a racecar on low octane fuel—it pings! You need iron to help oxygen reach all parts of your body; with little iron, you lack energy. If you've already gotten your period, you'll need even more iron because you lose it with the blood you lose each month.

This group is not without pitfalls, however. Being American is synonymous with eating which food? You got it—beef. And which member of this group has a lot of protein but also has the highest fat and cholesterol content? Beef again. As a country, the United States is technologically, medically, and economically advanced, but when it comes to nutrition, we are poor role models for the world.

> A cow needs to consume 21 pounds of protein in order to produce one pound of protein for us humans to eat.

Which country is a much better role model? The mainstay of the Japanese diet is rice, raw fish, and a lot of veggies, which are all naturally low in fat and rich in nutrients. This diet takes the health lead. Japanese living in Japan have a lower incidence of heart disease and breast cancer than Americans or than Japanese people born and raised in the U.S. Don't walk, run to your local sushi bar! Raw fish tastes much better than it sounds, I promise.

> Next time you're out on a boat and feel queasy, don't feel too embarrassed, even fish can get seasick.

Fish is not your only low-fat, high-protein option; there are eggs, beans, lentils, peas, and tofu. When it comes to meat, choose the leanest types and cuts, such as chicken or turkey, or beef's tenderloin and sirloin cuts. Every now and then, indulge. For me, what's a professional baseball game without a hot dog with mustard and sauerkraut? Oh boy, that's making me hungry; I've got to run to the fridge.

Okay, I'm back. Have you ever been curious about what it would be like to go **vegetarian** and eliminate meat altogether? Eating a vegetarian diet can be the most healthy way to go; the trick is to put the time and effort into replacing all the specific vitamins and minerals that you'd be missing. Some vegetarians include dairy and/or fish in their eating plans, while other people eat no animal products whatsoever (called **vegan** vegetarianism). If you're considering going veggie, you've got to take the responsibility seriously:

- Develop a nutrition plan with your doctor or professional dietitian.
- Read a couple of good books on the subject (I list a few at the end of the chapter).
- Take vitamin supplements that your doctor or dietitian recommends.
- Have fun by experimenting with ethnic cuisines that make vegetables interesting and delicious.

> For veggie lovers there's a lot of unexplored territory: Of the 80,000 known edible plants, we humans only grow 300 of them. But don't go picking around your backyard—that could kill you.

If you're eating meat and fish, then here are a few fun, healthy options.

### ACTION: The Iron and Protein Round-Up

1. **Popular Healthy Foods:** Have a protein boost with eggs for breakfast (but not every day because the cholesterol adds up). For lunch? How about tuna that comes packed in water, with pickle relish for pizzazz (but light on the mayonnaise), stuffed into a whole wheat pita pocket with lettuce and tomato. For lunch

or dinner, try lentil soup, vegetarian chili, or a vegetarian burrito. For a snack, peanuts, pistachios, almonds, or sunflower seeds.

2. **The More Exotic Route:** Be adventurous; I hear that ostrich tastes like red meat, yet has less fat than chicken. Give this big bird a try. But if the words "big bird" bring up images of a yellow childhood friend of yours on *Sesame Street*, you may want to skip it. Around the world, people eat unusual animal meat. Eating turtle in the Bahamas was a yummy experience for me until images of my first pet ever, Pee Wee the teeny tiny turtle, floated into my mind. In Africa, I declined an offer of snake. I wasn't in the mood, but people said it was quite good.

3. **Quick and Easy Recipe: Hummus Spread (creamed chickpeas) from the Middle East**

What you need:
   1 can of chickpeas (save the liquid they come packed in)
   1 tablespoon lemon juice; either squeezed from a lemon, or from the bottle will do
   ¼ teaspoon fresh pressed garlic or garlic powder
   2 tablespoons tahini (sesame paste) or sesame seeds
   1 whole wheat pita bread

What to do:
   Put all the first four ingredients into a blender or food processor, blend until smooth.
   Cut pita bread into pieces shaped like slices of a pie.
   Dip the bread into the spread. (Try dipping raw carrot sticks as well.)

---

Ostrich eggs are the largest in the world at six to eight inches long. A single egg would take forty minutes to hard-boil, or would produce 11½ omelets.

**Fats, Oils, and Sweets Group**: A popular parental warning is "No sweets before dinner." It's no wonder they say this: sugar is the *only* food that fills you up with calories, but doesn't provide any nutrients. Cookies before dinner means that you won't have much room left for nutritious food. Sugar is sneaky, though; it may work its way into your dinner anyway. Sugar is hidden in many foods, such as ketchup, peanut butter, and some crackers. (Maybe that's why so many of my cousins love ketchup sandwiches; it's a sweet tooth, not the mutant ketchup gene I thought they had.) Sugar also comes disguised in many different forms, including honey, brown sugar, molasses, maple syrup, and corn syrup.

Do you know which is the only form of sugar that comes packaged with nutrients? Fructose, which is found in fruits. Since your body needs *some* sugar for energy, why not go to fruits to get it? But remember, you don't want a candy bar for energy. Too much sugar will lift you up, oh so briefly, and then let you down hard, making you reach for your next quick sugar fix: A junk food junkie is born.

> A typical American kid consumes approximately three to four pounds of refined sugar a week, but only 36 percent of it is eaten directly; the rest is "hidden" in prepared foods that are commercially sweetened, like ketchup, cereals, and canned fruits.

Fat can be sneaky as well by swimming around in places you would least expect it, like salad dressings. Margarine still has the same fat and calorie content as butter. Also, if you cook highly nutritious foods, such as potatoes and chicken, in fats and oils, you zap the nutritional value right out of them—French fries and fried chicken are the result.

How do you handle the urge for sweets and fats so that they don't take over the entire food pyramid? The answer is simple: Indulge yourself sometimes; denying yourself only makes the cravings more powerful. If you yearn for sweets, don't feel bad—nature wanted it this way; you were born with a sweet tooth. Researchers found that newborns responded more quickly to sweet tastes than to bitter, sour, or salty ones. Here are some tips on how to bring sweetness into your life, along with good nutrition.

### ACTION: Sweet Health

1. **Wash Your Dessert Down with a Healthy Drink:** Have a glass of skim milk with your cake or apple juice with your pie.

2. **Substitute Fruit** (I love it when words rhyme): Want to sweeten up cereals or pancakes? Add pieces of fruit or fruit yogurt. Eat a fruit salad for dessert. If you need chocolate, make chocolate-covered strawberries or bananas.

3. **Experiment with Spices:** Put cinnamon on your French toast and nutmeg on your cereal.

4. **Be a Smart Consumer:** Try products that say "low-fat" and "low-sugar." Be a label sleuth; check out the ingredients listing for any form of sugar that may have been added. If they're listed toward the front, then you know that there's a lot of added sugar.

5. **Quick and Easy Recipe: Crunchy Banana Pops**

What you need:
>  3 recently ripened bananas
>  1 small container of your favorite flavor of low-fat yogurt
>  ½ cup crushed peanuts
>  3 popsicle sticks

What to do:
>  Mix up the yogurt in the container and then spread it out on a plate.
>  Add the peanuts to the yogurt.
>  Cover a cookie sheet with wax paper.
>  Unpeel the bananas and roll them one by one in the yogurt/peanut mix.

Set the bananas down on the wax paper and insert
a stick into each.
Cover with wax paper and put in the freezer until
frozen.

---

Sodas have been around for about 200 years, yet it was
only 100 years ago that they earned the name "soda pop";
the beverage was served in a glass bottle with a cap that
needed to be popped off, making the sound "pop."

---

## The Drink of Life: Water

All this talk about food, and we haven't even mentioned
what your body needs you to ingest in the largest quan-
tity—water. You might be able to survive for six weeks
without food, but without water, you wouldn't be able to
live for more than about a week. You are literally swimming in water right now—up to 70 percent of your total
body mass. Water is in your blood, your tissues, and even
your bones. Almost every body process takes place in a
watery medium; could you imagine chewing without saliva?

---

You don't just drink water—you eat it too. A large
percentage of most foods is water: 91 percent of broccoli,
84 percent of an apple, 71 percent of a baked potato, 65
percent of a skinless portion of roasted chicken, 37 percent
of cheddar cheese, and 38 percent of a slice of whole wheat
bread. It's no wonder we have to eat so much food to get
all the nutrients we need.

---

Water is elusive; you need so much of it, yet it's escaping from your body all the time. You don't have to be
perspiring or urinating to lose water—just breathing does

it. Oops . . . there it goes again. Rather than stop breathing, simply drink at least eight glasses of water a day, even more during the humid, hot summer.

Water is cost- and calorie-free; but what do Americans drink most? My guess is that coffee and sodas win out. This is unfortunate because the caffeine found in most of these drinks comes disguised as a hydrating liquid, but it actually drains your body of fluid so that you pee more often. So why did a friend of mine bring coffee with him on our week-long backpacking trip into the hot, waterless desert? Because caffeine can be addictive and he was addicted. I, too, was hooked once but broke free; caffeine was messing with my body's natural ability to stay awake and sleep when I needed it to. I've been decaffeinated and full of energy for years and highly recommend it.

---

The more water you drink, the more radiant your skin appears.

---

### ACTION: Keeping Your Body Well-Watered

1. **Drink Water All the Time:** Don't wait until you're thirsty to drink; thirst is your body's way of warning you that you're on your way to dehydration.
2. **Throw a Bottle of Water into Your Bag:** Take it everywhere, refilling it in the water fountain throughout the day. Drinking water in public gives you that healthy girl-on-the-go aura.
3. **Don't Worry About Tap Water:** It's safe and healthy. You can always use a filter if you prefer.
4. **Drink More When . . .** Being physically active or sweating in the summer heat requires a lot more fluids.
5. **Avoid Caffeine:** Opt for juice and water instead of soda, and herbal decaffeinated tea instead of coffee.

If you're already addicted to caffeine, then phase it out slowly to ward off possible withdrawal headaches.

6. **How Do You Know If You're Drinking Enough Healthy Fluids?** Your urine holds the answer: A small amount of intensely colored urine means that you need to drink more, while a good amount of pale-colored urine signals that you're well-watered.

7. **Incredibly Quick and Easy Recipe:** Mix fruit juice with sparkling water or seltzer and you get a drink with fizz and pizzazz.

---

In the U.S., approximately 700 different brand labels of bottled water are sold, including mineral water, sparkling water, spring water, well water, and sometimes even water from the same source as tap water. Remember to recycle those plastic bottles!

---

## Lifestyles of the Nutrient-Rich

When you think about drinking eight glasses of water and look at the food pyramid, you may be wondering, "How am I supposed to eat and drink all of that in one day? I'm a busy girl!" The great news is that whatever time you spend eating nutritiously is given back to you ten times over in the amount of energy you'll have to fuel your hectic day. But I bet that in the rush of life, you may miss a meal altogether. Am I right? If you said yes, I can look into my crystal ball and predict that you probably have an aversion to breakfast. Right again?

Then here are some facts you should know: By eating breakfast, you can join the cheerier, more productive morning crew, and improve your academic performance. Throw me all your excuses for not eating breakfast; I can field them.

- **"I'm not hungry in the morning—food is the last thing on my mind."** Your hunger may not have broken through into awareness, but trust me, your body is hungry, even if it's too tired to tell you so. Your body hasn't been fed for 8 to 12 hours. That's why the meal is called breakfast: break-the-fast.
- **"I think not eating breakfast is a good way to lose or maintain weight."** In the next chapter, I'll talk about how eating breakfast actually *helps* you stay slim!
- **"I don't have enough energy to eat at that time."** Eating *gives* you energy!
- **"I don't like the typical breakfast foods."** No problem, leftover macaroni and cheese, pizza, chicken sandwich, or soup are perfectly healthy choices. (One of my ketchup-loving cousins used to eat spaghetti with ketchup for breakfast.)
- **"I don't have time to eat."** Set your alarm for ten minutes earlier and grab a quickie breakfast like whole wheat bread with peanut butter, a glass of juice or milk, and an apple for the road.

Once you get over the hump and start eating the morning meal, you'll start to crave food in the a.m. and your stomach will ask for it with a growl. Here are a few more suggestions on how to make enough room for food in your life.

A government survey in 1995 found that half of all girls ages 11 to 19 were consuming less than two-thirds of the amount of nutrients they needed to fuel good mental performance and normal growth.

### *ACTION: Making Way for Nutrition*
1. **No Excuses for Not Eating Lunch Either:** If you find the mystery meat at the school cafeteria too much of a puzzle, then ask the cafeteria staff if they have

vegetarian meals stashed away in the back. Or bring your own meal in a brown bag or maybe a hip vintage lunch box. (Some girls even use lunch boxes as purses.) Devising your own sandwiches can be fun.

2. **Pack-a-Snack:** Snacking is the best way to keep yourself revved up all day long. So why did snacking get a bad name? It's probably because in the United States, snacks became synonymous with soda, potato chips, candy bars, and cookies. But you and I know that snacks don't have to come from the tippy top of the food pyramid. Pack healthy snacks like tiny cherry tomatoes, grapes which go "pop" in your mouth, or your own trail mix blend of nuts, raisins, and dried fruit.

---

On what day of the year do Americans eat twice as many snacks as they do on any other day? Hint, they're watching a nationally televised event.

The answer: Super Bowl Sunday. Maybe the bowl in Super Bowl represents a large bowl full of snacks!

---

## Confessions of Fast-Food Obsessions

Does eating according to the food pyramid seem pretty simple? If you answered, "Yes," then can you tell me why so many kids are way off the nutrition mark? Could it be because the fast-food chains—McDonald's, Burger King, Wendy's, Kentucky Fried Chicken, Taco Bell—are everywhere and lure kids in with their tasty foods, not to mention the toy giveaways? Here's my confession of fast-food obsession:

---

When children under age 17 eat out, they dine at fast-food joints 83 percent of the time.

Where I live in Greenwich Village, New York City, I'm surrounded by exotic restaurants, quaint cafes, and fast-food chains. For three entire years I walked past my neighborhood McDonald's and never looked back, until the day I started dating a guy who was hooked on McDonald's burgers and fries. When I'd accompany him around the corner to Micky D's, it was impossible to watch him eat those delicious fries and not grab a few for myself (you know what I mean). I soon found myself slowing down every time I approached the McDonald's, thinking, "Oh, those fries sure are good, no matter how greasy they are." It took all the willpower I had to keep on walking by. I even started having dreams about fries and I'd wake up in the middle of the night, wondering if the restaurant was open. Although my fry craving lasted longer than the boyfriend did, willpower won out; I eventually stopped dreaming of and yearning for fries.

---

During a nine-month period of daytime weekend TV viewing, a kid could have seen 3,832 commercials for breakfast cereals (many of them containing a lot of sugar), and 1,627 for candy and chewing gum, but only two advertisements for meat and poultry and one each for vegetables and cheese.

---

Why was the McDonald's fries habit so hard for me to kick? Because the fast-food restaurants have put a lot of research and money into making their food irresistibly greasy, sugary, and salty. You don't have to avoid the fast-food chains altogether, just eat smaller portions of the less nutritious foods; maybe have a small fries on the side or pour your milkshake into cups to share with friends. And definitely, make healthier choices once you're there. Here's how:

Why is it better to eat foods low in salt? Salt can leach calcium from your bones and contribute to high blood pressure. Besides, a lot of salt masks the subtle flavors of food.

### *ACTION: Avoid Becoming a Fast-Food Junkie*

1. **Add Nutrition:** Put lettuce and tomato on sandwiches, instead of mayonnaise. Heap veggies onto your pizza instead of sausage and pepperoni. Order a side order of corn on the cob instead of fries. Get the salad bar as a meal, or on the side, but watch out for the creamy dressings and pasta salads.

2. **Drink Well:** Have juice, water, or low-fat milk, instead of soda and milkshakes.

3. **Avoid the Greasiest of the Grease:** That goes for deep-fried foods with crispy coatings, or breakfast croissants and biscuits. If fried chicken is on your must list, then peel off some of the crispy skin.

4. **Let Lean Be Your Guide:** If it's red meat you really crave, then go to a Roy Rogers or Arby's outlet; roast beef is usually much leaner than a burger. Even a plain taco is better—less meat.

5. **Fast Health Food:** Take advantage of the following products when you see them: low-fat burgers, veggie burgers, broiled chicken, and baked fish.

6. **Go the Exotic Route:** Rather than sitting on a hard chair at Micky D's, you could be sitting on a cushion on the floor at a traditional Japanese restaurant. Rather than unwrapping the paper from your meal, you could be ripping off pieces of a giant communal pancake and using them to eat spicy Ethiopian dishes. Go for an eating adventure in your own town; there's Thai, Indian, Mexican, Italian, Middle Eastern, Polish, Vietnamese, Chinese, and don't forget regional American foods like Louisiana Cajun and more. Ethnic cuisines are often quite healthy.

There are 11 to 15 teaspoons of sugar added to your typical fast-food milkshake, no matter the flavor, and nine teaspoons added to a can of soda.

## Retraining Your Cravings

Are you tempted now to make a few changes in your eating habits? That's great if you are. Know, though, that it may take a little time to adjust, but the difference you'll feel is so worth it. Did you know that most of your food cravings, like your taste for fat and salt, were not with you at birth? They developed when you were exposed to salty and fatty foods. Anything learned can be unlearned; it just takes a little time. Let's say that you now have the goal of drinking skim milk instead of whole. At first the low-fat variety will probably taste bland and watery. But after two weeks, the skim will taste yummy, while whole milk will taste too rich, like cream. Give it a try and let me know if this happens to you. After you've made a few changes in your eating habits, take the nutrition quiz on my website, *www.TheGirlsGuides.com*, to find out how your efforts are paying off.

If you retrain a couple of your cravings, eat and drink a balanced diet, and get your groove on, then maintaining a healthy, trim weight should come naturally. But if you mess with your body's nutritional balance through dieting, you will likely put on extra weight in the long run. The next chapter relates other surprising dieting facts, along with my simple and fun six-point guide to a having a healthy weight.

## Check Out These Resources

### Phone numbers and Websites

American Dietetic Association
(800) 366-1655 (Regular weekday hours: Referrals to nutritionists and dietitians, plus advice.)
Website: *http://www.eatright.org*

Vegetarian Youth Network
E-mail: *VYNet@mhv.net*
Website: *http://www.geocities.com/RainForest/Vines/4482/ index.html*
Discusses vegetarianism and animal rights. Kids share recipes and meet pen pals.

### Books

Jacobson, Michael F., Ph.D., and Sarah Fritschner. *The Completely Revised and Updated Fast-Food Guide.* 2nd ed. New York: Workman Publishing, 1986, 1991.

Krizmanic, Judy. *The Teen Vegetarian Cookbook.* New York: Puffin Books, Penguin Group, 1999.

Larson, Roberta. *The American Dietetic Association's Complete Food and Nutrition Guide.* Chicago: Chronimed Publishing, 1996.

Pierson, Stephanie. *Vegetables Rock! A Complete Guide for Teenage Vegetarians.* New York: Bantam Books, 1999.

Salter, Charles A. *The Nutrition-Fitness Link: A Teen Nutrition Book.* Connecticut: The Millbrook Press, 1993.

# SEVEN

## Don't Diet—Lead a Healthy and Trim Lifestyle

In sixth grade, Cathy was a busy girl with schoolwork, marching band practice, and going to movies with her girl-friends. Eating heartily fueled her hectic days. She always ate what was given her for breakfast, lunch, and dinner, and then some—she snacked a lot. The number of calories in her food or pounds on her body never even crossed her mind.

Then, in seventh grade, the girls in Cathy's class started weighing in and reporting their scores; the two to three digit numbers they discussed were no longer their test scores but their weight. Curious now about her own weight, Cathy noticed the scale that had been gathering dust in the corner of her bathroom. She pulled it out, dusted it off, and stepped on board. She noted the number, but it didn't mean that much to her.

Pretty soon, many of her friends were pinching their stomachs and complaining about how overweight they were. Cathy thought they looked great as usual, but no amount of compliments could penetrate their self-dissatisfaction. Even Cathy's younger sister joined the "I'm too fat" club. Surrounded by girls who thought they were fat, when they were actually normal or even underweight, what was Cathy to do? What many girls do—Cathy started questioning her own perception of reality. "If they're over-weight, I must be pudgy too. Time to diet."

Cathy began weighing-in at least twice a day. She gave

her mother a list of the foods she would and wouldn't eat based on their calorie content. She was constantly checking out her stomach profile in the mirror and giving herself the waist-pinch test. Cathy had gone from happily weight-oblivious to unhappily weight-obsessed in a matter of weeks.

> More than 50 percent of girls ages 8 to 11 thought they were too fat and wanted to lose weight, even though most of them fell within the normal weight range.

Cathy no longer saw how beautiful she was. And what she certainly didn't know was that her scale lied to her and that dieting would make her plump. You must be thinking, "Scales lie? Diets *put on* weight?" In this chapter I will turn everything you thought you knew about weight loss upside down. In place of all the misinformation about weight that our culture promotes, I'll share with you the few simple do's and don'ts I live by that have kept me as fit and trim as I've wanted to be.

Luckily, my secret six-point plan happens to be backed by scientific evidence and involves being a hearty eater who's happy with her body. I hope to initiate you into the Female Eats Club—together we can show the world that girls and women can strengthen themselves through food, rather than weaken themselves through deprivation. The first step is to take the Lifestyles of the Slim and Trim Quiz to determine what you're already doing that's on the right track.

*Quiz:*
*Lifestyles of the Slim and Trim*

1. When it comes to dieting:
   a. I never diet or I tried dieting and don't plan do it again.

    b. I'm on the lookout for the next miracle weight-loss product or plan.
    c. I always seem to be on one weight-loss regimen or another.

2. When it comes to exercise:
    a. I love exercise and do it regularly.
    b. I exercise when I have time or exercise sometimes because I should.
    c. I avoid exercise at all costs.

3. I eat:
    a. When I'm hungry.
    b. At the regular meal times.
    c. When I'm hungry, sad, nervous, or bored.

4. My weight and the calorie content of food:
    a. Aren't things I think about or I've been told by a doctor to pay attention to them, so I do.
    b. Are on my mind sometimes.
    c. Guide most of my food choices.

5. When it comes to eating:
    a. I eat three big meals and snack rarely or I snack a lot and eat smaller meals.
    b. I don't have regular eating habits.
    c. I skip whole meals on a regular basis.

6. When I'm feeling full after having eaten a lot, but not all, of my dinner:
    a. I stop eating.
    b. I play with the food until I'm hungry again and then finish it.
    c. I finish what's left anyway.

7. When I eat:
    a. I chew slowly, savoring the flavor, and enjoying the conversation.

b. I eat fast or slow depending upon how many other things I have to do.
c. I eat quickly, and sometimes don't chew my food very well.

**Scoring the Quiz:** An (a) response = 1 point; (b) response = 2 points; and (c) response = 3 points. When you add up your total for the quiz, if your score falls between 7 and 11, then you're Stylin'; between 12 and 16, then you're Stumblin'; and between 17 and 21, then you're Sinkin'.

**Stylin':** You must be a natural when it comes to trim living. Your body has a rhythm that keeps you on the move and well-fed, and you follow it. Read on to understand why what you're doing works. You might also pick up a few more tips along the way.

**Stumblin':** Your instincts about healthy living are pretty good, but sometimes you have trouble following them. Learn where you're on track and where you've taken a detour. If a fit and trim lifestyle is what you're after, then it's right at your fingertips.

**Sinkin':** Somewhere along the line you've fallen out of step with your body's natural rhythm. The tips in this chapter will help you get in touch with what your body needs to maintain its healthy weight. No major life makeover, just a few easy changes; you'll probably even enjoy making them.

---

Among girls ages 8 to 11, 43 percent have already made attempts to lose weight. Most females who begin dieting start between the ages of 8 and 13.

---

Before learning about my six-point plan, find out the real facts behind America's dieting culture.

# Dieting Makes You Plump, Not Skinny

I've never dieted, but if I had, I would probably be pudgy now. You know those ads that show women before and after they went on the diet plan? Well, if there were truth in advertising, the "after" shot would show the women a few months later back at her old weight or even heavier. The human body's response to rapid weight loss is to put the pounds back on again as quickly as possible, and then add some. If the person tries to diet again, then it's harder for her to lose weight and the pounds come back on even more quickly. This is called the "yo-yo dieting effect"; up and down and up and down.

---

Here are the yo-yo dieting facts: Ninety to 98 percent of people who diet regain all or more of any weight they may have lost. For example, if somebody loses 100 pounds through dieting, she usually gains back 125 pounds, making her heavier than when she began.

---

Here's how it works: If you go on a diet, restricting the amount of food you eat, your insides scream, "Famine is coming!" This sends all systems into emergency mode. Your body does whatever it takes to keep a healthy amount of meat on your bones:

**You Become a Pantry Closet.** Your body grabs hold of whatever food you do eat and stores it as body fat, which then serves as an emergency source of energy.

**Your System Goes on a Slow-Down Strike.** Since you're feeding your body less fuel than it needs to function properly, it tries to use less energy. To conserve, your metabolism (the rate at which all your basic functions run) slows down so you need less fuel to breathe, eat, walk, talk, sleep, and simply have your heart beat. When the diet ends, the rate at which you burn your incoming food is still slower than normal. It's a speedy metabolism that helps you stay trim.

> Small animals have faster metabolisms than large ones. A hummingbird must eat all the time or else it will die from starvation within hours, while the blue whale can survive without food for up to half a year by living off of its blubber.

## Dieting Makes Your Life Worse, Not Better

Ads for weight loss portray perky, happy, skinny women. A truthful ad would depict women who are tired, irritable, and ill. Here's what dieting, weight-loss aids, and pills may do to you:

**Mess with Your Development.** Stunt your height growth and prevent menstruation.

**Mess with Your Mind.** Make you moody, depressed, and feel like a failure.

**Mess with Your Energy Level.** Render you inactive; with less nutritional fuel, you exert yourself less. Inactivity is a huge risk to your weight and health.

**Mess with Your Health.** Give you stomach pains, nausea, and fatigue, not to mention heart, kidney, and liver problems, and painful gallstones (like little pebbles going through your internal system).

**Mess with Your Lifespan.** Possibly kill you. For example, if you take diet pills, your body develops a tolerance, meaning that it takes more and more pills to get the same effect. Girls have easily overdosed this way and died. Another example is the popular low carbohydrate/high protein diet which denies your body an important energy supply, forcing it to cannibalize (literally eat itself alive!) all your lean body tissue, which includes your heart, liver and other organs.

---

A low-calorie liquid diet popular in the 1970s, called the Cambridge Diet, was advertised as "the perfect food." Thirty people died from it before the FDA made it illegal.

---

## Scales Tell Lies, Not Body Truths

Your scale pretends to be your best friend, patiently waiting in the bathroom until you honor it by stepping on board. You ask, "Oh scale, oh scale, on the floor, do I need to lose more?" It reliably answers you with a number. But what it doesn't tell you is that this number is misleading because:

**Muscle Weighs More Than Body Fat.** Muscle tissue is mostly water and protein, making it heavier than fat tissue. So, since exercising regularly strengthens your muscles, you'd probably appear thinner while weighing more. It's no surprise then that two girls can be the same height and 35 pounds apart in weight, yet both be within the healthy weight range.

**Your Weight Can Vary from Day to Day.** Depending upon your clothes, shoes, and how much liquid and food waste you're retaining, your weight will fluctuate within a small range of pounds. That's why you will weigh more right before you get your period each month—bloating.

---

The 208 bones that structure your body weigh 20 pounds.

### ACTION: Being Hip to the Hype

1. **Don't Be Suckered.** When you see an ad for a magical weight-loss regimen or a friend tells you about these new dieting pills, recall what you now know about dieting; say "No."
2. **Spread the Word.** Let friends and family in on the real story behind America's dieting culture.
3. **Put Your Scale Out to Pasture.** Chant "Oh scale, oh scale, on the floor, you are no more!" and toss it out the window into the garbage can (I can't think of a charity to donate it to, can you?). A scale out of sight means pounds off your mind. Let your doctor be your weight-watcher at your regular check-ups.

> Home scales didn't become popular until dieting became popular in the 1920s. Before then, people went to drugstores and county fairs to weigh themselves.

So with the scale tossed and the diets ditched, let's get down to business. The following six-point plan will be the most fun guide to being fit and trim that you will find, or your money back (just joking about the money-back guarantee; I couldn't resist imitating those phony weight-loss commercials). You are already quite familiar with the first tip—exercising—but I promise a few surprises ahead.

### #1: Shake Your Booty

Ask any health professional what's the best way to maintain a healthy weight and they'll all likely give the same answer—exercise. How does exercise work its magic? Let me count the ways:

*Exercise, oh exercise,*
*You make me feel so good that I don't need nibbles*
*to be merry*
*Exercise, oh exercise,*
*You create muscles where there once were none*
*Exercise, oh exercise,*
*You set my metabolism racing for hours and hours*
*Exercise, oh exercise,*
*You burn food as fuel*
*Exercise, oh exercise,*
*You make me feel healthy and strong*
*Exercise, oh exercise,*
*I need you.*

---

What percentage of the girls in your class exercise on a regular basis? Only 30 percent of girls in their first year of high school regularly exercise vigorously, and half of the girls who do exercise, stop by the time they graduate.

---

### ACTION: Maximizing Your Moves

1. **Find Your Groove.** Discover an activity you love and you're set. Aim to do it three to four times a week for an extended period (at least 30 minutes).
2. **Shake More than Your Booty.** Aim to give all your muscles, including your arms and legs, a workout. I do the walk-dance; if you ever find yourself in Greenwich Village and see a petite woman wearing a Walkman and waving her arms, bobbing her head, and moving her legs to her private beat, that would be me.
3. **Don't Become a Fitness Freak.** Exercising all the time, every chance you get, is bad for the body. It needs time to rest and restore itself between workouts. I can think of two activities that are healthy for

you to have the urge to do all the time—smiling and laughing. Are there others I've missed?

**4. Couch Potatoes—Sprout Some Legs.** Next to sleeping, watching TV is as inactive as your body can get. So,

**a. Break that hypnotic trance.** Turn off the tube and do something else, anything else—more power to you. Of course, every now and then, a complete veg-out in front of the tube is a must.

**b. While watching:** Stretch; put a puzzle together; knit; or do what I used to do, make jewelry. In high school, I turned my TV-viewing and phone-talking into a thriving jewelry business. Who knows what you'll create? During commercials and in between favorite shows, say hi to your parents or take the garbage out. If you miss part of a TV show, you can play the game of trying to guess what happened before you tuned in; it gets you to at least exercise your brain while watching.

---

Kids in a study who were encouraged to watch less television put on less body fat after a six-month period.

---

### #2: Eat Small Amounts Often

Want to keep yourself revved up to exercise and be trim? The best way to do this is to eat small amounts of food often throughout the day, while avoiding stuffing yourself during the big three-meal feast. This will give you constant energy, as well as keep your metabolism running at high speed. Not to mention the fact that you'll be less likely to overeat in one sitting because your body won't be craving a ton of food.

There's an official term for eating often: **grazing**. It's too bad that grazing most often gets associated with which animal? The cow, which is generally considered large and lazy. The official mascot of grazing should really be the slender deer—a runner and a grazer. I've lived the grazing lifestyle for years and it has worked well for me. People have been astounded at how often I eat and yet, don't put on weight. I'm proud of my Female Eats approach to life because it shows the world that we women can nourish, not starve ourselves.

---

A study of moderately overweight women found that those who ate breakfast actually lost more weight than those who skipped breakfast. Why? A good breakfast prevents you from grabbing something quick and fattening later in the morning and keeps your metabolism running up to speed.

---

### ACTION: Successful Grazing

You may be thinking, "Since I'm not a deer and there are no fields around for grazing, what do I do?"

1. **Pack a Snack.** Buy a box of those handy-dandy Ziploc bags and pack snacks. When you bag your own portable nibbles, you can create a variety of healthy choices and determine your own portion size, which prevents mindless grazing in the field. When your parents see you putting together your own healthy snacks, they'll do a double take. And don't forget to pack the bottled water; I know that drinking the recommended eight glasses every day helps keep my hunger at just the right level for my body.

2. **Don't Be a Meal Martyr.** Try not to go more than five hours without eating something.

3. **Listen to Your Hunger.** Get to know your early hunger cues. Is it a stomach growl? Or do you imagine that you keep smelling a hot dog, but there's no hot dog in sight? Then, when your body asks for food, you can feed it. What if you nibble all day and aren't exceedingly hungry for the big dinner your parents serve? No problem, read on . . .

Companies have found that the more employees snack, the more they work, so many bosses supply closets or carts full of snacks.

### #3: Doggie-Bag It

I advise giving your parents advance warning that you've resigned from the Clean Plate Club and have joined the Doggie-Baggers. You enjoy their food, but you don't want to eat it all at once. I'm a notorious doggie-bagger when I eat out: I've bagged on first dates, bagged on the way to a party and temporarily left it in a stranger's fridge, and I've been known to bag it with just four bites left. Challenge me—there isn't a doggie bag opportunity I'd be too embarrassed to take. Believe it or not, some hot foods even taste better cold—like my Jewish mom's delicious homemade lasagna.

### ACTION: Joining the Doggie-Baggers Club

1. **Listen for When You're Full.** How do you know you've had enough? The food on your plate no longer looks appetizing? Your stomach feels heavy? Learn your various satiety signals and obey them.
2. **Say, "That's a Wrap."** If there's still food on your plate, but you're no longer hungry, there's power in being able to stop and say, "That's a wrap."
3. **Bag It, Box It, Tupperware It:** Keep it in the fridge until homework time or lunch tomorrow.
4. **Reminders.** Draw pictures of the food on sticky notes to remind yourself that the food is hiding in the fridge; out of sight tends to be out of mind.

### #4: Eat Slowly

What helps you find your stopping point? Eating slowly. Eating slowly eases digestion and gives you the chance to feel when your stomach is getting full. Did you know that your stomach can be full for 20 minutes before it lets the brain know? I call this dysfunctional communication between stomach and brain.

---

In the late 1890s a popular "chewing" diet called for at least 20 chews per mouthful of food.

---

I . . . eat . . . sooooooooo . . . slow . . . ly;   I   have   no choice. If I eat quickly, I feel queasy. I eat so slowly that friends who have finished their meal try to sneak food off my plate and waiters lurk nearby, waiting to snatch the whole plate away. This forces me to institute plate defense; I keep my fork in my hand and look busy. But this strategy doesn't always work. If anybody invents a plate protector gadget, like a force field or a plate alarm, I would be forever grateful.

### ACTION: Slowing Down

1. **Savor Every Bite.** Allow all the subtle flavors to register, and take a break before the second helping; you'll be better able to tell if your stomach wants more. Wouldn't it be cool if there were a line of foods that changed from one luscious flavor to another with each chew? That would certainly be an incentive to chew longer.
2. **For Those of You in a Large Family.** Is dinner like a free-for-all of food-grabbing and gulping down? Then slowing down will be quite a challenge. Start the meal by putting a good-sized portion on your plate. And if I hear of a good plate protector, I'll let you know.
3. **Chat.** Enjoy the company at the meal. Speak your mind in between bites (but after you finish chewing, of course).

Have you ever stopped to wonder what type of music they play in the background at fast-food restaurants? Often they play fast music as a way to get you to eat quickly and move on out. That's also why the seats are hard—they don't want you to get comfortable. Several McDonald's in Washington, D.C., posted signs warning "No Loitering. 20 minute time limit consuming food."

### #5: Eat Your Food, Don't Count It

To help you on your mission to savor your food and eat more slowly, don't count calories or fat grams; simply enjoy what you eat. Food was made to taste delicious and we humans were given taste buds on our mouth and tongues with which to savor it. If all food tasted like raw lima beans, we'd all stop eating and die of starvation.

Tasting food depends on more than just taste buds. You need saliva, a sense of smell, and the sense of touch inside your mouth related to temperature. Try putting salt on your dry tongue—you'll taste nothing. Try holding your nose when you bite into an onion—it'll taste sweet like an apple.

There's no one particular food in and of itself that has the power to make you fat. If so, this food could have served as a great nonviolent wartime strategy—send this fat-bearing, irresistible food to the enemy troops; they'll gobble it down and become so sluggish that their only option is to surrender.

You could go to a family brunch, where you eat bagels with heaps of cream cheese and lox, French toast, and coffee cake. Then you could go to a friend's birthday party that evening and snack on bowls of M & M's and Cheez Doodles, have two slices of pizza, soda, and chocolate cake with an ice cream sundae. And the next day, you'd be back to your old weight. Overeating for a day won't make any difference. You would have to overeat for a period of a couple of weeks, without adding any extra exercise, to put on a pound of body fat. Your body wants desperately to maintain its set point weight. So enjoy your day of food gatherings and return to your healthy balanced diet the next day.

### ACTION: Eat and Enjoy!

1. **No Guilt or Shame Allowed.** So dig in. Eating is pleasure. Simply try to respect the wisdom of the sacred Food Pyramid as often as you can.
2. **If You Overeat One Day.** Just return to your regular diet the next.
3. **Ignore the Calorie Content.** When it comes to calorie counting, I'm proud to report that I am absolutely, positively clueless. In this case ignorance is bliss because knowledge equals obsession.
4. **Don't Panic.** If you accidentally stumble upon the calorie content of a food and notice a really high number, don't worry. The one thing I *can* tell you about calories is that they usually come packaged in the double or triple digits.

---

In the 1880s, Midwestern towns passed laws prohibiting the sale of ice cream sodas on Sunday. Creative soda fountain owners got around the law by leaving out the carbonated water and serving just the ice cream and the syrup. Hence the name "Sunday soda," which was later shortened to "Sunday" and then, "sundae."

---

### #6: Know Your Foods from Your Moods

Have you ever felt anxious about schoolwork, so you finished a whole bag of potato chips and the rest of the ice cream carton while studying? Or felt really sad about an argument with your best friend, and eaten the whole pan of brownies between bursts of tears? Don't kick yourself for indulging a mood with a food; everybody does it. The problem comes in when you feel ill because you're eating when you're not really hungry. Plus, once you're done eating, the bad mood still lingers.

### ACTION: Sorting Out Food and Mood

1. **Is It Your Head or Your Stomach?** Where is the activity in your body at that moment? Is your head swimming or your stomach or both? A stomach rumbling means food is in order. A head spinning should put you on mood alert. If you have both, then it could be a sign that your mood has led to a nervous stomach.

2. **Mood Management.** What do I recommend when you're feeling down or upset or bored? When I'm in a bad mood, I do two things:

a. **I jump-start** myself into a better mood by talking to a friend, going for a walk, writing a poem in my journal, or doing a physical activity.

b. **I use my Thought Tracer Technique** to figure out the source of the mood. You can do this too by asking these questions:

- When did this feeling begin? Five minutes ago? An hour ago?
- What was going on at the time? What was I doing? What was I thinking about?
- When you hit that trigger thought, a "ding" will go off in your head. Examine that thought rationally; Is such a small thought worthy of creating such a big bad mood? If your answer is no, your mood will likely perk up. If your response is yes, then tackle the problem head-on. Are there ways you can overcome the obstacle? If the problem is out of your control, like your parents are fighting a lot, consider finding a professional to talk to (see page 246) and write in your journal in the meantime.

3. **Loss of Appetite.** If a bad mood can take away your

hunger for more than a few days, ask yourself if you're feeling very sad, sluggish, and worthless, and either sleeping too much or too little. If so, then you may be slipping into a depression. See Chapter 10, pp. 244–253 on seeking help and regaining your happiness and your appetite.

The last tip isn't part of the official plan, but it's the most important.

## Be Nice to Yourself

There's no being hard on yourself in my plan. Nobody follows a new lifestyle plan perfectly, so give yourself a break. My suggestions are just that, mere suggestions. You can decide to put them into action now, years from now, or never. You are being armed with knowledge, so any action you take is icing on the cake (thought I'd use a nondieting metaphor).

A health expert said that it's easier to get people to change their eating habits than it is to get them to exercise. Do you agree or disagree? What's been easier for you—following the advice in the sports chapters or the food chapters? Let me know; we can do our own girl poll.

> Will your stomach shrink if you eat less? Nope. It can expand temporarily to accommodate more food coming in, but then it returns to its normal size once the food passes through.

## It's Fitness, Not Fatness, That Matters

Are you convinced now that dieting is dangerous, and that there are better ways to stay slim? Maybe you've wondered at different points in this chapter, "But isn't being extremely overweight dangerous too?" Cutting-edge researchers are finding that people who are slightly overweight but who also eat well and exercise regularly may actually be healthier than people who are at an average weight but don't take good care of themselves. While exercising is possible for obese girls, they unfortunately are less likely to engage in physical activities because the extra weight on their bodies requires more exertion. This means that many girls who are highly overweight are actually at high risk for heart disease, high blood pressure, diabetes, and cancer.

Obesity has multiple causes, including genetics. How can you know whether or not you are seriously overweight, especially when every other girl in America thinks she weighs too much? Odds are that you're far from overweight, but the following action will help you gain a quick assessment and tell you what to do.

### ACTION: The Obesity Question

**1. Take the Unofficial Alice-in-Wonderland Quiz: Does the World Seem Too Small for You?**

a. Do you have trouble fitting into a one-seat allotment on the train or bus?
b. Do doorways seem too narrow?
c. Are clothes big enough to fit you extremely difficult to find?

If you answered yes to any of these questions, then you may be dangerously overweight; if so, read on.

**2. Ask Your Doctor.** If your doctor determines that your weight is jeopardizing your health, then, with her or his assistance, devise a fitness and nutrition plan. Nobody should attempt to lose weight without following a doctor's advice.

Do you know what's special about May 5? It's not
Mother's Day (close though). It's national No Diet Day,
organized by the National Association to Advance Fat
Acceptance.

## When Girls Are Dangerously Thin

Some girls are naturally underweight and find that gaining
weight isn't all that easy. Maybe they're born with an extra-
speedy metabolism or maybe their brain signals to them
that they're full when they're not. Without enough food-
energy, these girls tend to get tired, irritable, and have trouble concentrating. The origins of being too skinny are
complex; genetics play a role. If you find that you're
super-skinny and you don't know why (i.e., you haven't
been trying to lose weight; you don't have an eating disorder), here's what to do.

### ACTION: Putting Some Meat on Your Bones
1. **Eat According to the Higher Servings of the Food
   Pyramid.** Stay within the guidelines, just on the
   higher end.
2. **Eat Often.** Definitely be a grazer.
3. **Drink Fluids 30 Minutes Before and After Meals,
   Not During.** Beverages fill you up; so leave more
   room for food.
4. **Stimulate Your Hunger.** Keep your favorite foods
   handy. Take a brief walk before mealtime.
5. **See a Doctor.** Don't wait to wither away—consult a
   doctor and professional dietitian. Get some meat on
   your bones; this isn't just your grandmother talking.
   If you are experiencing a sudden rapid weight loss,
   this may be a symptom of another problem that needs
   medical attention.

## Wrap-Up

Can I deem you a new official member of the Female Eats Club? Will you help me show the world that not all girls and women count calories and pounds? If our revolution succeeds:

> Scale makers will have to find another product to manufacture (what could it be?).
>
> Restaurants, even fast-food joints, will have long lines of people waiting outside, while you girls take your own sweet time eating.
>
> Households will need bigger refrigerators with special little drawers to accommodate all the doggie bags.
>
> Schools and communities will have to add more girls' sports programs and teams!

Maybe you have your own healthy slim-living tip you'd like to add—let me know and I'll tell the girls on my website. There's one dieting danger that I saved for last; when dieting gets out of hand, eating disorders can take over. Are there any aspects of your life that increase the odds of you developing an eating disorder? The next chapter will let you know and tell you how to protect yourself.

---

Eighty percent of people with an eating disorder started with a diet.

---

Americans spend a total of $30 to $50 billion every year on weight-loss plans and gimmicks that do not work.

# Check Out These Resources

## Phone Numbers and Websites

Shapedown
(415) 453-8886 (Regular weekday hours, charge for call:
   Referrals for adolescent obesity programs.)
E-mail: *shapedown@aol.com*

General crisis counseling: Kid Save Hotline: 1 (800) 543-
   7283 or National Runaway Switchboard: 1 (800) 621-
   4000.

*www.healthyweightnetwork.com*: The Healthy Weight Network brings you the latest scientific information on nutrition and maintaining a healthy weight, and helps you
   apply it to your life.

*www.beyonddieting.com*: This site discusses and encour-
   ages healthy lifestyle choices.

*zaphealth.com*: This site provides information for teens on
   sex, drugs, alcohol, mental health, family problems, skin
   problems, weight issues, and sports injuries. You can ask
   an expert for advice.

## Books

Barrett, CeCe. *The Dangers of Diet Drugs and Other
   Weight-Loss Products (The Teen Health Library of Eating Disorder Prevention)*. New York: The Rosen
   Publishing Group, Inc., 1999.
Drohan, Michele Ingber. *Weight-Loss Programs: Weighing
   the Risks and Realities (The Teen Health Library of Eating Disorder Prevention)*. New York: The Rosen Publishing Group, Inc., 1998.

# EIGHT

# When Dieting Gets Out of Hand—
## Eating Disorders

What is wrong with this picture? In college, my boyfriend, who claimed to have dated only fashion models before dating me, told me that I should stop eating bagels because my behind was too big. At the same time, my boss, a world-renowned family therapist who had specialized in eating disorders, kept expressing his concern that I was so dangerously thin I must be anorexic. A boyfriend who wanted to get me to Weight Watchers and a psychiatrist boss who wanted to get me to an eating disorder clinic—I promise you, I did not make this up.

So what happened? If I had listened to the boyfriend, I might have started a diet that could have turned into self-starvation, and then my boss would have *had* to check me into a clinic. Fortunately, I listened to my own hunger and kept on eating healthily as I always had. The boyfriend? He decided that he liked intellectual women—big brains became more important to him than butt size; he fell into a depression when I broke up with him. The boss? One day we ate lunch together and he was shocked that I ate more than he did.

Clearly, our society is messed up about body size if I could be told at the same time that I was overweight and dangerously underweight. This chapter is designed to help you understand what may put you at risk for an eating disorder and how to protect yourself. This topic deserves at least a whole chapter because you, my reader, being a female in your preteen to teen years are more at risk than anybody else for developing eating disorders.

---

The age at which girls are most likely to start developing an eating disorder is right at the time of puberty, ages 12 to 15, but it can be as young as seven or eight years old. Girls with eating disorders outnumber boys by at least nine to one. In response to an increase in body image pressures on males to be muscular, the rate of male eating problems is on the rise.

---

I want to reassure you that just because you may have finished a whole bag of potato chips, a giant Coke, and the leftover cake while watching a movie one evening doesn't mean that you have a problem controlling your eating. And just because you had a nervous stomach for a few days and ended up picking at your plate doesn't mean that you are in danger of starving yourself. It's perfectly fine to raid the cookie jar once in a while and to pick at your plate every now and then. But destructive patterns can develop quickly. This next quiz will help you determine whether or not you're currently in the danger zone.

## Quiz:
### Are You in the Danger Zone?

1. When I sit down for a meal:
   a. I'm extremely nervous because I'm convinced that whatever I eat will make me fat.
   b. I avoid certain foods because I fear they'll make me overweight.
   c. I enjoy the taste of what I eat.

2. When I eat sweets and salty snacks:
   a. I can easily get way out of control and eat whole boxes and bags full of different foods all at once.
   b. Sometimes I find it hard to stop snacking once I start, but in general, I'm in control.
   c. I generally eat small amounts at a time.

3. I exercise:
   a. Vigorously, as often as I can in order to burn off the calories that I eat.
   b. On a regular basis in order to maintain my figure.
   c. When I feel like it to have fun and feel healthy.

4. When it comes to dieting:
   a. I've already tried different plans and am always searching for the perfect diet.
   b. I've thought about dieting and haven't done it yet, but I may in the future.
   c. I know that dieting is not for me and I don't plan to diet in the future.

5. After I finish eating dinner, I leave the table feeling:
   a. Either still very hungry *or* so overly full that I feel fat.
   b. Either slightly hungry *or* full and slightly bloated.
   c. Pleasantly full and satisfied.

6. My weight is something:
   a. I think about *all* the time, even though people don't think I'm overweight.
   b. I think about occasionally and measure every so often, even though people think I'm skinny.
   c. I rarely consider, *or* I keep an eye on because I've been told that I'm unhealthily over- or underweight.

7. When it comes to food, what I pay most attention to is:
   a. Exactly how many calories it has.

   b. Whether the food is considered "bad" junk or "good"
      health food.
   c. How healthy and yummy it is.

8. When I finish eating a big meal or a lot of food:
   a. I feel guilty and vomit, take a laxative, or do what-
      ever it takes to get rid of the food in my stomach.
   b. I feel guilty and have contemplated getting rid of the
      food but never have.
   c. I feel pleasantly satisfied.

9. My family:
   a. Is extremely concerned about my eating and always
      tells me to eat more than I do.
   b. Is beginning to worry that I don't eat enough.
   c. Doesn't have any concerns about how much I eat.

**Scoring the Quiz:** An (a) response = 1 point; (b) response
= 2 points; (c) response = 3 points. When you add up
your total for the quiz, if your score falls between 23 and
27, then you're in the Safe Zone; between 16 and 22, you're
in the Danger Zone; and between 9 and 15, you're in the
Serious Trouble Zone.

**In the Safe Zone:** You are living what this book is all
about: having healthy attitudes about food, weight, and
your body. This chapter will help you hold on to these
feelings in the face of whatever challenges the future may
bring. There may be certain aspects of your life, such as
family troubles or school pressures, that put you at risk for
developing dangerous eating behaviors. In this chapter, you
can identify these risks and learn how to safeguard your
life against eating disorders as well as increasing your happiness quotient.

**In the Danger Zone:** You are living on the borderline between an eating disorder and healthy habits. You may be
thinking, "Who, me?" The problem is that trying to do

things that control your weight can quickly take control over you, becoming a deadly addiction. Pay close attention to this chapter—it could save your life. It will help you understand why weight and food are becoming an issue for you and give you ways to move yourself into the safety zone. After you finish this chapter, I recommend another quick read through the "Don't Diet" chapter.

**In the Serious Trouble Zone:** You are losing control over your eating. You may be like many girls with eating disorders: a high achiever who got sidetracked by food issues. This chapter will help you understand why food has become such a battleground for you and guide you toward health. The longer an eating disorder continues, the harder it is to conquer. If you don't conquer it, it will conquer you. Seeking help from an adult you trust or a doctor on your own initiative is an admirable move that requires strength and maturity; I know you can do it.

---

Experts agree that eating disorders are very dangerous, but what they can't agree on is the percentage of American teens who suffer from them. Estimates go as high as one out of every ten teens for a full-blown disorder, and one out of five for occasional dangerous eating behaviors. To save you the math, this means that in a class of 15 girls, three are likely to have eating problems.

---

If after taking the quiz, you're thinking of skipping this chapter, you should know that this chapter is chock-full of helpful advice on how to handle life's stresses—everything from parental pressure to teasing from classmates.

## What Is an Eating Disorder?

Here's a brief description of the many ways eating troubles express themselves:

**Anorexia:** Fear of becoming fat leads to gradual self-starvation—a slow form of suicide.

**Bingeing:** Eating a huge, tremendous, gargantuan amount of fatty and sugary food (e.g., a jar of peanut butter, a box of doughnuts, a pint of ice cream, and a box of sugared cereal) within several minutes to a couple of hours.

**Purging:** Getting rid of food after it's been eaten by vomiting or taking a laxative (a pill that induces a bowel movement).

**Bulimia:** A combination of bingeing and then purging afterwards.

**Binge eating disorder:** Eating a very large amount of food in one sitting often; over time, this leads to obesity.

**Exercise addiction:** Exercising excessively with the goal of burning off all the calories that were eaten.

**Combination:** Many of the people who fall into one of the groups listed above also engage in behaviors from the other groups. For example, a large percentage of anorexic girls engage in excessive exercise.

---

Do you know which eating disorder is one of the fastest-growing? Exercising to lose weight has become a dangerous obsession for many since the beginning of the fitness boom two decades ago. It can lead to severe weakening of the body and even death. If you are exercising several times a day to lose weight, then turn to the sections at the end of this chapter and book for seeking help.

---

I was hesitant to relate all this information because studies have found that simply educating girls on the nature of eating disorders can actually put them *more* at risk for developing one. But I have faith in you that you will use the information I give you wisely; you have chosen to read a book on how to be good to your body, not harm it.

# Dr. Foodenstein and the Monster

An eating disorder often begins when a girl tells herself she just wants to lose a little weight. She feels the need to take control over at least one part of her life or to be "perfect" in every way. But too often, a split second of taking control flips and the girl is on her way toward having an eating disorder take over her life. Of course, when a girl first begins dieting, bingeing, or purging, she doesn't say to herself, "Today I'm going to start an eating disorder," but unfortunately that's what happens. The eating disordered behavior grabs hold of her and won't let go. You've heard of Dr. Frankenstein, who created a monster that also came to be known as Frankenstein, who then tried to murder the doctor? It's the same here; the girl with an eating disorder is like a Dr. Foodenstein, who creates the monster Foodenstein (an eating disorder), that's determined to destroy its creator.

Girls who have survived or are struggling with eating disorders can describe it best. Survivors have opened up to authors of various books. You'll hear from these girls, as well as from a couple with whom I spoke myself.

> Kelly:
> *Once you start bingeing, it's like cigarettes. It's a hard habit to break. It's with you for years, maybe even a lifetime. You think you can stop any time, but your fear of getting fat is so overwhelming that you're driven to this extreme behavior.*[10]

> An anonymous former anorexic:
> *I was in so much pain, I didn't think I had any other options. I was caught in this eating disorder and just watching myself slowly committing suicide.*[11]

> Among college women, 80 percent reported being
> "terrified" of being overweight.

## How the Foodenstein Monster Destroys

It's not just a girl's mind that loses control, it's also her body. You've already learned about how your body can function well when you feed it well, so I'm sure you can imagine how the body reacts when the nutritional balance is thrown way off. Now add the violence done to the body through repeated induced vomiting or use of laxatives.

> Brenda was trying to stop purging, but found that she would vomit even when she wasn't trying anymore:
> *I can't stop . . . it just happens. It's only supposed to happen when I make it happen. Will I even be able to eat and digest again?*

> Kelly, who suffers from bulimia:
> *One afternoon, I was sitting in traffic school and suddenly I got this tingling feeling in my hands and then my muscles started contracting and curling up and contorting. My whole body froze! I excused myself and went to the pay phone to get help and when I started walking back, I screamed, "Oh, my God!" and I collapsed on the floor by the classroom—my legs were paralyzed. I couldn't move any of my muscles, even my tongue! . . . The doctor examining me told us I had had a minor heart attack.*[12]

Eating disorders damage most of the body, including the brain. A heart attack isn't the only cause of death, there's also the rupturing of the stomach or esophagus, sheer starvation, or depression leading to suicide. Not to mention all the medical complications, such as severe weakness and fainting spells that make everyday living a nearly impossible task. Can you see why I'm so concerned?

---

The percentage of people with an eating disorder who die as a result of the illness may be as high as 20 percent—one out of five.

---

## What Puts You at Risk and What Protects You

There are certain aspects of your life that make you more vulnerable to developing eating disorders (these are **risk factors** or **stressors**) and other aspects that strengthen you against developing them (**protectors**). I can tell you for certain that you definitely have two risk factors: your age and your sex. This is a vulnerable time in your life when your body is changing, along with the social scene around you. On the positive side, I can reassure you that you already have two protectors: the guidance of this book and the fact that you're obviously interested in learning how to take the best possible care of your body. What are your other risks and protectors? Take the checklist test to find out.

## The Risk Factor Checklist

There isn't enough room to list every possible risk factor, but these should be enough to get you thinking. Do you struggle with the following stressors? Check "yes" or "no" for each.

**YES   NO**

____ ____ I'm an athlete, dancer, or model and therefore experience pressures to be a certain weight.

____ ____ I have an athletic coach or instructor who emphasizes body size and shape.

____ ____ My parent is concerned about her or his own weight, or the weight of other family members.

____ ____ My friends are always talking about how they don't like their bodies the way they are.

____ ____ Classmates, my parents, or siblings have teased me about my weight or body shape.

____ ____ I feel pressure to date or to go further sexually with a guy than I want to.

____ ____ I have been sexually or physically abused by somebody.

____ ____ My parents like to take over the decisions in my life.

____ ____ My parents don't get along with each other or are separated/divorced.

____ ____ I have a stepparent or two.

____ ____ My family and I have moved to a different part of the country from where I grew up.

____ ____ I feel pressure to be perfect in my schoolwork and in all other ways.

____ ____ My parents aren't around much.

____ ____ I feel like a failure.

____ ____ I believe that foods are either "good" or "bad" and that I'm good or bad depending on what I eat.

____ ____ I go on diets.

____ ____ I'm unhappy with how my body looks.

____ ____ I feel sad and weepy quite often.

____ ____ Somebody I know well has an eating disorder.

____ ____ One parent (or both) abuses alcohol and/or drugs.

____ ____ I watch a lot of TV and read magazines.

How did that go? It's not easy to face the troubles in your life, even if it's just on paper. When you count up the number of stressors (all your "yes" answers) and protectors (all your "no" answers), how do they balance out? The presence of even just a couple of stressors, especially in the absence of protectors, could mean that you're at high risk for developing eating disorders, or even other troubles, such as depression or alcoholism. These next few sections on family, friends, and more will help you better understand the stresses in your life and build up protectors against them.

---

What happens around February 14? Sure, there's Valentine's Day, but there's also National Eating Disorder Awareness Week. Be on the lookout for it.

---

## Coping With Stresses and Creating Protectors

**PARENTS**: Parents hope to be your protectors in life, and often are. But sometimes, parents are so overwhelmed by the stresses in their own lives, like marriage and job problems, that they end up stressing you out too. Does that sound at all familiar? Girls who suffer from eating disorders often have struggles going on inside their families. As they speak of their difficulties, listen for issues that might ring true for you.

Anonymous:
*I wasn't allowed to make any decisions for myself. I thought, if I can't be trusted to make one little decision, I must be a total loser. My weight was one area of my life that I had control over. No one could make me eat if I didn't want to.*[13]

Emily:
*You could say I had a normal appetite until my
mom remarried. . . . He isn't that nice to me. But
then sometimes he is. It gets confusing. Anyway,
after their wedding I start[ed] to overeat. In the
beginning I guess I [did] it out of anger about the
whole situation. Things are really tense around
the house. Like, my stepfather makes these so-
called jokes about charging me rent, and that I'll
probably still eat more than I can pay him. Every
weekend I go to my dad's. Now he's married to
a woman named Miranda. She looks like she
could be a model, and to go along with that, she's
always on a diet. My dad tells me, "Fat people
are disgusting. Be thin. Be beautiful. Miranda will
teach you how to diet." So I diet with Miranda,
and I sneak extra food when I'm alone.*[14]

Heather:
*It's my parents. My mom calls Dad the Shadow
Man. He's never home. She thinks he's running
around. She says she doesn't have enough money
to get a divorce. I'm totally upset and just can't
eat.*[15]

Catrina, looking back on her time in high school:
*Years later I discovered what I had not known
about my family—that at the time of my anorexia
my mother had discovered that my father was
having an affair. I had always wondered why neither my mother nor my father seemed to notice
that I only weighed 70 pounds! I believed that they
didn't love me enough to care whether I was
healthy or unhealthy, whether I lived or I died. In
retrospect I realize that they were too caught up
in their own problems to focus on my weight
loss—perhaps I tried to distract them from their
own difficulties, but instead it only made things
worse for all of us.*

Parents of girls with eating disorders may also have a misguided approach to eating. It can be quite confusing for a girl when parents encourage dieting, not knowing how unhealthy and ineffective it really is. Also, if your mother or sister has an eating disorder, then be on extra alert—you've got a double whammy of genetic risk and a home life that makes dangerous eating behaviors seem normal.

Parents who are able to be consistently loving are definitely the best source of protection against eating disorders for their daughters. Yet even with amazing parents, girls may develop eating problems.

When life at home is rough, everything else can seem rough too. Give yourself a break—family troubles are difficult for any kid in your situation. The following suggestions can help you cope if you're struggling at home all the time or even just occasionally.

---

Of these choices, which do you think the majority of girls are most afraid of: losing their parents, a nuclear war, getting cancer, or becoming fat? Becoming fat was the top fear. What would you answer?

---

### ACTION: Coping With Rough Family Situations

1. **It's Not Your Fault!** First and foremost, I want to state that whatever—I repeat *whatever*—is going on with your parents, is *not* your fault. For example, if your parents argue about how to discipline you, it's just an excuse for them to disagree; their strife has nothing, zero, to do with you or your sisters and brothers.

2. **Free to Be You.** If you feel like your parents aren't around much or are trying to control your life and pressuring you, try to carve out areas of your life in which you can express and assert yourself. Speak up in class more, join a club or debate team, write short

stories, or gather a group of friends who cherish you. Form a special relationship with a teacher, the librarian, or an older cousin who can help give you the appreciation you deserve.

3. **Getting Parents' Positive Attention.** Wishing your parents would pay more positive attention is a good wish. Here are a few suggestions on how to try to make your wish come true, but don't blame yourself if your efforts aren't effective.

a. **Tell them what you miss** about them when they're not around.

b. **Suggest fun things** you can do together.

c. **Ask for their opinions** on something you're doing for school.

d. **If they're running an errand**, ask if you could come along.

4. **Parents Are Imperfect.** You want to love and admire your parents, yet sometimes they make you upset. When you have a negative thought about your parents, do you feel guilty? You shouldn't. You are not betraying them when you think to yourself, "I wish they wouldn't do that." Allow yourself to feel your hurt. Right now, list in your head or on a piece of paper, what you admire about your parents and what you wish they would change.

5. **Weight Control.** If parents are recommending that you alter your eating habits, let them know that you are struggling to feel good about yourself the way you are and have been reading up on dieting dangers. If they say that they're more concerned for your health than for your appearance, ask them to go with you to discuss the weight issue with a doctor.

6. **Talk with an Adult.** If the situation at home is very stressful, seek professional help by utilizing the resources lists and last chapter of this book. Getting the support you need is not betraying your family, it's helping them; ultimately, what your parents want most is for you to be happy, even if they don't always do a good job of expressing that.

**FRIENDS AND CLASSMATES:** Have you ever been with a bunch of girls who get onto the topic of their bodies and weight? It's unfortunate how they can be so hard on themselves. This is the type of atmosphere that sparks competition for who can be the thinnest and smallest; in other words, who can be the first to disappear, as if disappearing is an accomplishment.

> Anonymous survivor:
> *I had to be the best at everything I did. If there was a test, I had to get the highest grade. If girls were going to diet, I had to be the thinnest.*[16]

Have you ever felt swept up in the tide of insecurity? Or has the tide of insecurity turned against you, such that kids teased you about your body? These situations could put you at risk for eating disorders. It's easy to feel, "If I just lose weight, then I'll be accepted." The sad, awful irony about eating disorders is that they usually make a girl feel incredibly isolated from everybody around her:

> Pilar:
> *In my mind, I started purging to lose weight so that I would be more attractive and, as a result, be more popular and worthy of others' interaction. But what resulted was that I wasn't able to interact at all. It became impossible to keep this "secret" and be with people at the same time.*[17]

> Nicole:
> *I stopped going anyplace I wasn't certain I'd be able to use a bathroom in private. I wanted to hang out with friends, but I couldn't. The bulimia came first, before anything.*[18]

Does anybody you know have an eating disorder? I ask because just knowing somebody, whether a close friend or an acquaintance, who is suffering from anorexia or bulimia actually increases the odds that you might develop the disorder. There's a temptation to copy the eating behavior, especially because these girls are often perfectionists and high achievers. But they're paying a high price with their eating disorder, including low energy, brittle bones, and depression. Remind yourself that they're accomplished and admirable girls despite their eating disorder, not because of it.

Are your friends bashing their bodies, or is somebody putting you down? Here are some tips on how to cope.

### ACTION: Coping with Tough Situations

1. **Redirect Your Friends.** If you're immersed in a group of girlfriends who are stuck on fat talk, try to unstick them. Invite them over for a mystery video festival, play soccer, play a bunch of board games, hold a talent show, take silly pictures of each other, rewrite the lyrics to your favorite songs, or do something crafty—like beaded jewelry or painted T-shirts—they'll love this! If your girlfriends can't go beyond body, then it's probably time to go beyond this group of friends and find new ones.

2. **Stop the Teasers.** Kids who tease want to appear tough, so nobody will know how insecure they really are and pick on them. If these kids truly knew you, they'd be begging you to be their friend. To fight back:

a. **Enlist the help of an adult**, whether it be a parent, a teacher, a school counselor or principal, or a religious leader. (If you witness teasing, ask an adult to intervene.)

b. **Come up with a creative counterattack.** When I was seven, a boy at school pulled my hair and called me names every day. Adults weren't of much help to me, so I took matters into my own hands. I followed him around all day and repeated the word "frog" over and over, driving him nuts. More than a year of teasing took one day to extinguish. Be inventive. If you have any suggestions for other girls, send them my way; I'll post them on my website: *TheGirls-Guides.com.*

---

When kids as young as two years old were shown dolls of different body types and asked which dolls have the most friends, they answered, "The thin ones do." It's good that skin color and the presence of a physical disability, such as being in a wheelchair, didn't make a difference. But it's troubling that our culture teaches children that weight matters.

---

**COACHES OR ACTIVITIES THAT HAVE WEIGHT REQUIREMENTS** can put tremendous pressure on girls to do unhealthy things to their bodies. If you're an athlete or performer, you know what I'm talking about.

> Nicole, who suffers from bulimia, said that she didn't think she was overweight until she joined her school's gymnastics team:
> *That first week of practice a lot of girls had aching wrists or knees. The coach sat us down to say, "There's a lot of pounding in this sport. Some of you—and you know who you are—have excess baggage that you're throwing around, and it isn't going to help those sore joints that you've got."*[19]

### ACTION: Dealing with Weight Pressures

1. **Get Parents Involved.** Have a meeting with your parents and the coach to discuss how unhappy the weight requirements are making you. Coaches sometimes don't realize the pressure they inflict.
2. **Consult a Doctor.** If the coach still insists that you lose weight, consult a doctor first on whether or not this would be healthy for your body and if so, do it

under supervision of a professional nutritionist, doctor, or dietician.

3. **Switch Teams.** Consider joining a community team or a different sports team. Remember, you shouldn't do and die for your team; coaches don't always know best.

---

Which group of women has the highest rate of eating disorders? Professional athletes, followed by women in the military.

---

**SELF-ESTEEM:** With pressures from school and from home, it can be difficult to keep your self-esteem intact. Most girls get down on themselves sometimes, but some girls always feel that they aren't worth much. Does this sound like you? If I asked you right now what you think of yourself, what would you say? If you answered anything less than "I'm a terrific person," then there's work for you to do on building up your self-esteem. Did you know that almost all girls with eating disorders have low self-esteem?

> Peggy, a mom, describes her daughter, Kirsten:
> *Sometimes she would look at some minuscule bite of food on her plate and tell me, "Mom, this hurts so much. I shouldn't be eating it. I should be eating a quarter of it. That's all I deserve." She felt almost subhuman, less than the rest of us. She never knew why she was less deserving, but she just knew she was.*[20]

> Anonymous survivor:
> *I thought all of the bad things that had happened in my life were my fault. I didn't know it at the time, but I was punishing myself—by starving myself and making myself throw up.*[21]

If you have low self-esteem, then you use any mistake you make as proof of your inadequacy. Other people would just toss it off as a mistake, but not you. If you're trapped in perfectionism, any positive feeling you have about yourself just slips right through your fingertips. The ultimate in feeling worthless is feeling like you don't deserve to live; a very large percentage of girls with eating disorders are also battling depression. High self-esteem is the most powerful defense against eating problems or any major disorder. Here are a few pointers for getting to know how lovable and special you truly are.

> In today's media, many of the actresses, models, and beauty pageant contestants meet the weight criteria for anorexia.

## ACTION: You Are Great and It's Time You Knew That

1. **Pat Yourself on the Back.** Congratulate yourself for reading this book and wanting to make your life the best it can be.
2. **Come to Your Own Defense.** Write down all the bad thoughts you have about yourself. Next, make arguments against each. For example, maybe you're thinking, "I'm so stupid. I can't do math to save my life." But you're forgetting about how well you did on that English exam last week. So you're not dumb; it's simply that you find some subjects harder than others, just like everybody else. Think of yourself as a defense lawyer who represents good causes, such as this one—the defense of yourself against all the bad thoughts in your head.
3. **Bring in Witnesses for Your Defense.** If you have trouble coming up with counterarguments, solicit evidence from others. Believe me, other people generally see us much more positively than we see ourselves. In high school I thought I was extremely

shy and boring; but it turns out that many people saw me as outgoing and witty. So trust yourself, except when it comes to the disparaging thoughts you have about yourself—then become suspicious.

4. **Examine Your Standards.** The high standards you set for yourself, where do they come from? From parents, or competition with a sister, brother, or friends? Do you expect more from yourself than you do from your friends?

5. **Celebrate Imperfection.** Rejoice in the fact that neither you, nor anybody else, is 100 percent perfect. Think about your friends and their quirky imperfections; aren't these part of what you love about them?

6. **Be Active.** Participate in activities that make you feel good about yourself. Just learning something new is worth self-congratulations. Take music or photography lessons. Take a book out of the library on how to paint with watercolors and give it a try. Volunteer to help others with your skills or give some tender loving care to abandoned pets at the pound. (See the website for resources on how to explore your potential.)

---

Store mannequins are so thin that if they were real women they would have only ten percent body fat. In order for females to menstruate regularly, they need to have *at least* 17–22 percent body fat.

---

**BODY IMAGE:** The majority of girls who develop anorexia or bulimia start off at near average weight, yet see themselves as fat anyway. In striving to look like the "thin ideal," these girls wind up looking incredibly unhealthy. Girls with bulimia typically stay at or close to their normal weight, but their teeth decay from the acid in their vomit and their cheeks often puff out. For girls struggling with anorexia, their bones and ribs start to stick out and their arms and legs end up looking like toothpicks. Their clothes size often dwindles down to children's sizes, but when they look in the mirror, their brain tricks them into seeing a size 14.

These girls often look at the way the media portrays females and think that being skinny is the ticket to popularity. In actuality, the majority of males are *not* attracted to females who are dangerously underweight. It doesn't make biological sense for a male to be drawn to a female who has lost so much body fat that she cannot menstruate, and thus, cannot reproduce his genes. Here's a real conversation that my 13-year-old friend Maggie and her pal Fred had when a skinny girl walked by:

Fred: Ooh, that girl is *so* skinny.
Maggie: Isn't that what guys like?
Fred: No. I like a girl with some body on her.

Here are a few reality check tips:

### ACTION: Fighting the "Thin is In" Message

1. **Synonyms for "Thin."** Look up "thin" in your thesaurus. What do you find? I found that although skinny and lean were listed, most of the words were hardly complimentary: starved, emaciated, gaunt, haggard, wiry, bony, and scrawny.
2. **Less Media/More Activity.** If only you could turn on the TV or open a magazine and see girls and women the way they really look in the streets, in your homes, and in school. But since you often can't, exercise your option to shut off the TV or close up the magazine, and do an activity. Be physically active with a sport, exercise your imagination with art, or be politically active.
3. **Accept the Challenge.** Are we females going to let our culture kill us with media images?
4. **Reread the Chapter on Body Image.** That chapter is my protective offering to you.

In Fiji, a South Pacific island, a traditional compliment was, "You've gained weight." But since the introduction of Western television—and images of tall, slender women that come along with it—eating disorders are now on the rise there; they were practically nonexistent before. The girls who watched more television were also more likely to describe themselves as "too big or too fat" and to diet than the girls who watched less TV.

**FOOD:** Food is designed to be your life support, but in a culture of dieting, food can become your worst enemy. You overhear a friend saying, "I'm awful; I ate a whole bag of chips." Or maybe you see an advertisement showing a woman who ate an ice cream sundae and started on a diet plan the next day. Or maybe a parent gives you the message that certain foods should be avoided:

> Barbara, a survivor, recalling when she was seven years old:
> *Mom put me on a diet. I was chubby—not fat— and I couldn't bring dessert to camp with my lunch. I was the only kid with no dessert—every- one else had fun things. In my head, I was the fat kid who couldn't have things that other kids have.*[22]

Have you ever thought that the carrots were "good" and cake was "bad," and that you were good or bad depending on what you ate? Though these thoughts are common, they're also incorrect and extremely dangerous. By denying herself so-called "bad" foods, a girl creates intense cravings that can lead to bingeing on those very same "forbidden" foods. Feelings of guilt follow, which can lead to purging— bulimia. Or maybe all foods come to be seen as evil, as if one cookie or potato could lead to a 40-pound weight gain; this leads to avoidance of all foods—anorexia. Here are some ways to counteract the notion that foods are "good" or "bad."

### *ACTION: Don't Deny Yourself*

1. **Eat Your Favorite Foods.** Don't cut fatty sweets out of your eating altogether; simply eat these foods sometimes, and fruit and nutrient-rich snacks other times. Balance your diet according to the food pyramid so that you get all the nutrients you need. (Unless of course, your doctor advises against sugary foods because of a health condition, such as diabetes.)

2. **Take Normal Sized Portions.** When you do take a piece of cake, take a slice not a sliver. If you take a sliver, you'll still be denying yourself. Often one sliver can lead to another sliver and yet another, until most of the cake is eaten. Enjoy your slice of cake!

3. **Find Additional Ways to Treat Yourself Well.** Take long baths, give yourself a manicure, listen to music—do whatever it is that makes you feel pleasantly indulgent.

4. **Review Chapters.** Reread the nutrition and non-dieting chapters as a reminder of how you can eat well, maintain a healthy weight, and still enjoy food.

5. **Ask Yourself:** "If eating sugary and fatty foods really means that somebody is bad, would there would be any good people left in America?"

---

At what stage of your life do you require the most food per pound of body weight? You've been there already—as an infant eating day and night. Mothers who are breast-feeding should have T-shirts that read "Open 24 Hours." Because you're still growing now, you need more food than your parents do.

---

**ABUSE:** Any kind of abuse, whether it be physical hitting or shoving, sexual touching, or verbal criticism, can make a girl feel incredibly out of control. Even just one incidence of physical or sexual abuse can make the world seem like a dangerous place. Too often a girl who is abused blames herself for the attacks, despite the reality that only the abuser is to blame.

Feeling helpless and bad about herself can lead to feeling depressed, even suicidal; eating disorders may be one way that these emotions are expressed. If a girl has been sexually abused, she may use an eating disorder to try to make herself less sexually attractive to her abuser or to males in general. She may also be attempting to reassert control over her body.

If you have ever been abused in any way, by anyone, there are professional counselors ready to help. Abuse leaves emotional scars on everybody it touches, even though these scars are not visible to the eye. Just as a doctor heals physical scars, a counselor can help heal the emotional ones.

> When compared to women who were not struggling with an eating disorder, women suffering from bulimia were twice as likely to have a history of being raped, sexually molested, or physically assaulted.

## ACTION: Getting the Comfort and Help that You Need

1. **Why It Feels Hard to Seek Help.** You must get the courage to seek help, even if the person abusing you is someone you love or has warned you not to tell anybody. You need protection, and in the end, anyone who loves you will be glad that people intervened to help stop the out of control behavior.
2. **Getting Help Immediately.** If you are being abused now or have been in the past, no matter how long ago, turn right now to the resources at the end of this chapter, and the chapter on seeking help (page 244).

**DENIAL:** When an experience is too painful to face, a girl's bad feelings, and sometimes even her memory of what actually happened, are pushed underground, into the back recesses of her mind. These ignored bad feelings don't go away; the unhappiness grows and grows, but she can't understand why. These confusing emotions can express themselves in a variety of ways, including eating disorders.

> Anonymous survivor:
> *On the outside, I was the perfect little girl. On the inside, I was angry at my parents. But perfect little girls can't get angry, so I turned all the anger against myself.*[23]

At any time during this book when I described problems girls have, did you think to yourself, "That sounds like me"? But then a few seconds later, you thought, "That's definitely not me"? This means that part of you recognized the struggle you face, but another part of you found it too scary to admit; the result—denial. Don't feel bad; most people find it difficult to face their troubles head-on.

But I'm sorry to say that the only way to get painful emotions and memories to stop their destruction is to come face to face with them, no matter how difficult this may be. If your whole family tends to deny uncomfortable feelings, then it will be especially hard for you to unravel your emotions. Remember that denial increases the negative effect of all risk factors, such as family problems, because it pushes your awareness of them underground; how can you fight what you can't see? Here are a few ways to break any walls of denial that you may be building up.

---

Self-mutilation, in which a girl cuts or burns herself on a regular basis, is another way girls physically hurt themselves. Girls self-mutilate to feel something when they feel numb, or to punish themselves when in reality they've done nothing wrong. If you have thought of hurting yourself in any way, it's important to get professional counseling help immediately (see the chapter on getting help, p. 244).

### *ACTION: Denial-Busting Strategies*

1. **Cry.** Feel your sadness and let the tears stream down. Research has found that releasing teardrops actually makes you feel better. It can be scary to cry and feel as if once you start, you won't stop. But you will, I promise.

2. **Be Angry.** Stomp around your room. Throw some pillows against the wall. Take deep breaths, and then calmly let the people you're angry at know how you feel. It will be easier for them to hear what you have to say if you use "*I*" as opposed to "*you*" statements. For example, "I feel really upset when you tell me how bad my grades are" is better than, "You're awful for always criticizing me."

3. **Think and Analyze.** Write in a journal. Take a long walk to clear your head. Talk to somebody you trust or even into a tape recorder; simply expressing your thoughts and feelings can help. Also use the Thought Tracer Technique described on page 175.

4. **Speak with a Counselor.** See the chapter on getting help, page 244, for guidance on finding counseling. In my view, every one of us can benefit from at least a little therapy, no matter how big or small our troubles might seem.

---

Human beings are the only animals that cry.

---

## Triggering Experiences That Can Set Off an Eating Disorder

Often, but not always, a girl has a specific "triggering" experience that sets the whole pattern of dangerous eating behavior in motion. Here are particular experiences that survivors recalled:

- A girl walked by her dad, who swatted her hip with his newspaper and said affectionately, "Hey, you're getting kind of porky."[24]
- "My mom criticizes me, saying, 'A girl your size shouldn't be that heavy.' "[25]
- "My boyfriend says, 'If your stomach didn't stick out so much, you'd be sexier.' Then he dumps me."[26]
- A girl went to her doctor, who told her she was a little heavy for her height, but assured her she would grow out of it: "When I went home I wasn't thinking about it too much until my brother started teasing me, calling me a bowling ball. I went to sleep that night thinking about my weight and what I should do about it." The next morning she skipped breakfast, and so it began.[27]

People who make negative comments don't necessarily have malicious intentions, yet their words can have powerful effects. As you'll recall, my college boyfriend triggered me with negative comments about my buttocks, yet I didn't develop an eating disorder. Why not? First of all, I had protectors to counter the stressors in my life. Second, I had some suspicion of why the boyfriend said what he said. Considering that he kept telling me, "You're twice as smart as I am," he probably felt intellectually insecure in our relationship. He tried to comfort himself by making me feel insecure about my body. By figuring out where his criticism was coming from, I was able to lessen the negative impact of his words.

A comment about your body, a seductive ad for a dieting technique, overeating and feeling ashamed are all possible triggering experiences. Have there been any in your life? How have you handled them? The best way to stand strong is to remind yourself of what you like about your body and personality, and then examine the motivations of the trigger puller.

### *ACTION: Countering a Triggering Experience*

For each source, I offer one possible motivation behind the triggering. See how many others you can come up with:

- An advertisement for a weight-loss program or exercise equipment (wants you to buy their product).
- Your sibling (s/he wants to set you off).
- Your mother (she's uncomfortable with her own body).
- Your father (he's uncomfortable with your budding womanhood).
- A friend (she's jealous of your body).
- A boyfriend (he likes you so he's nervous and doesn't quite know what to say).
- A coach (s/he wants the team to win at all costs).

---

Eating disorders used to be virtually unheard of in China; overweight people were envied because of their assumed prosperous life. But now with the Chinese economic boom, anorexia and bulimia have multiplied dramatically in the past few years.

---

## What to Do if You Think You Might Be Developing an Eating Disorder

The first big step is one you've already begun to take—acknowledging that you have a problem. The next is asking for help. Many girls with eating disorders feel adamantly that they can take care of themselves, that they don't need any help. Unfortunately, once the addictive food behavior takes hold, overcoming it takes the assistance of many people, whether you're 12 years old or 40.

A survivor:
*Recovery is the hardest challenge I've ever had—*
*the hardest thing I've ever had to do. Recovery is*
*a choice. This choice is hard, but I don't want to*
*exist in hell, like I did before. I want to live.*[28]

You will never feel 100 percent certain (maybe not even 50 percent) that treatment is what you want, but you have to seek assistance. Getting help isn't just about getting rid of the hazardous eating patterns; it's also about learning to feel good about yourself.

### *ACTION: Getting Help*

1. **Setting the Help Team in Motion.** Utilize the resources listed at the end of this chapter, and read the chapter on Seeking Help, page 244. Give yourself a lot of credit for acknowledging that you need help and for taking the steps to get it; this takes true strength.
2. **The Treatment Team Might Include Several of the Following Helpmates:**
- A therapist who specializes in eating disorders
- Another therapist who meets with you and your family together
- A doctor who treats whatever medical problems you might have developed
- A nutritionist who can get you back on the healthy eating track
- A group of girls who also struggle with eating disorders
- A psychiatrist who, if necessary, could prescribe antidepressant medication, which has been shown to be very effective for eating disorders when combined with therapy
- A massage or acupuncture therapist, or maybe a yoga, meditation, or relaxation class
- A hospital stay might be required if the situation is life-threatening

The number of Americans affected by eating disorders has doubled during the period between the 1970s and 1990s. The biggest increase was among females between the ages of 15 and 24. Researchers connect this disturbing trend to the finding that, while in the 1970s only six percent of teenagers worried about their weight, in the 1990s that number had risen to at least 40 percent, and even higher for just girls alone.

## When You Suspect That Someone You Care About Has an Eating Disorder

Somebody else's health is not and cannot be on your shoulders. To get better, she will need a whole team of professionals trained in eating disorders. You can try sharing your concerns with your friend and also with adults who can set the help team in motion. But keep reminding yourself that only when somebody *wants* to change can anyone really help her.

> Noelle talking about her friend who has anorexia:
> *I wanted to help her live, not wait for her to die. I tried to make her eat. I tried to convince her she wasn't fat. She waved me away. I finally realized only she could make the difference; she had to help herself.*[29]

> Catrina:
> *My cousin Dave had approached me to tell me how "disgustingly skinny" I looked. Soon after, my best friend Susan called my mother to share her concern about me. I responded to Dave and Susan similarly by yelling at them to mind their own business! Nevertheless, years later, the two*

*people I feel most thankful for having had in my
life at the time are Dave and Susan—they helped
save my life and I've told them so.*

## Standing Strong

Rather than disappearing into bathrooms to purge or making yourself so skinny that you disappear altogether, you
and all girls need to unite and stand strong. You can show
the world what girlpower is all about; standing up for who
you are and asking for help when you need it. That is true
strength.

Being good to your body means not only feeding it well,
but also avoiding substances that can cause it harm, namely
tobacco, alcohol, and drugs; that's what the next chapter is
all about.

## Check Out These Resources

### Phone Numbers and Websites

Renfrew Center
(800) RENFREW or (800) 736-3739 (24-hours: Provides
referrals to local eating-disorder counselors, as well as
general information.)
Web site: *http://www.renfrew.org/*

National Association of Anorexia Nervosa & Associated
Disorders (ANAD)
E-mail: *anad20@aol.com*: Ask them questions.
Website: *www.anad.org*: To learn more about eating dis-
orders.

General crisis counseling: Kid Save Hotline: 1 (800) 543-
7283 or National Runaway Switchboard: 1 (800) 621-
4000.

*http://www.something-fishy.org/*: A lot of information on eating disorders and body image.

*http://www.gurze.com*: To order from their list of books on eating disorders, such as Liza F. Hall's *Perk! The Story of a Teenager with Bulimia.* (You can also call them at: (800) 756-7533.)

*zaphealth.com*: This site provides information for teens on sex, drugs, alcohol, mental health, family problems, skin problems, weight issues, and sports injuries. You can ask an expert for advice.

## Books

Chiu, Christina. *Eating Disorder: Survivors Tell Their Stories (The Teen Health Library of Eating Disorder Prevention).* New York: The Rosen Publishing Group, Inc., 1998.

Hornbacher, Marya. *Wasted: A Memoir of Anorexia and Bulimia.* New York: HarperCollins, 1998.

Kolodny, Nancy J. *When Food's a Foe: How You Can Confront and Conquer Your Eating Disorder.* Boston: Little Brown and Company, 1992.

Kaminker, Laura. *Exercise Addiction: When Fitness Becomes an Obsession (The Teen Health Library of Eating Disorder Prevention).* New York: The Rosen Publishing Group, Inc., 1998.

## Movie

*The Best Little Girl in the World.* Dir. Sam O'Steen. Perf. Charles Dunning and Eva Marie Saint. 1981. (A picture-perfect teenager hides her chronic anorexia from her family and friends.)

# NINE

## Keep Your Body Safe from Harm—Smoking, Alcohol, and Drugs

Susan is getting books out of her locker and Trish strolls by, "Hey, Susan, come hang with us at my house Friday night. Eight o'clock. Be there or be square." Before Susan can even respond, Trish is gone. Susan's grin takes over her entire face as she thinks, "Wow! I've finally been invited to hang with the popular people. Pretty cool. What to wear?" Her brow wrinkles—this is an important question to ponder. "Well, what do they do at these parties? Wasn't Maria saying something about dancing? R-rated flicks? Smoking and drinking?"

Susan frowns as she thinks, "Smoking and drinking. I've never done any of that before. They'll know what a loser I am." Then she recalls her parents' warnings of the dangers of alcohol and pictures the images from the D.A.R.E. video at school of nicotine's effects on the lungs. She snaps out of her nervous trance with the thought, "Hey, I'd just be trying it to see what it's like. And besides, they know what they're doing. They've been doing this forever. What's the big deal?" She closes her locker decidedly. But the books nearly fall from her hands and her stomach feels queasy. And so the internal struggle begins.

For every thought Susan has, there's a "But . . ." thought to go along with it. What would you advise her to do? What would you do in this situation? Alcohol and drugs are a complex issue. Some kids use them and seem to be fine.

Other kids use them and end up in way over their heads and sometimes even dead. Adults with a cigarette in one hand and an alcoholic beverage in the other tell kids not to smoke and drink, yet substances often wreak havoc on adults' lives as well. Alcohol and cigarettes are illegal for youth, yet there are beer commercials with croaking frogs that seem designed to appeal to kids. How are you supposed to make sense of all this? I'll do my best to help you sort it out. Let's start with a quiz to find out where you're at right now.

---

Why do alcohol and tobacco companies try to target youth even though it's illegal for kids to drink and smoke? The payoff is big. For example, if a beer company manages to hook a college freshman on their brand of beer, then that person will spend approximately $50,000 (with the effects of inflation figured in) to purchase the beer over a lifetime.

---

## Quiz:
### Cigarettes, Alcohol, and Drugs

1. When it comes to smoking:
   a. I either never tried smoking or did and disliked it—
      I plan to avoid smoking altogether.
   b. I've never tried smoking but would if I had the opportunity.
   c. I smoke every now and then.
   d. I smoke at least weekly or daily.

2. When it comes to alcohol:
   a. I either never tried drinking or did and disliked it—
      I plan to avoid drinking altogether.
   b. I've never tried alcohol but would if I had the opportunity.
   c. I drink occasionally.
   d. I drink at least weekly or daily.

3. When it comes to drugs:
   a. I either never tried drugs or did and disliked it—I plan to avoid drugs altogether.
   b. I've never tried drugs but would if I had the opportunity.
   c. I do drugs occasionally.
   d. I do drugs at least weekly or daily.

4. My friends:
   a. Are not at all into smoking, drinking, or drugs.
   b. Are curious about trying cigarettes, alcohol, or drugs.
   c. Smoke, drink, or do drugs every now and then.
   d. Smoke, drink, or do drugs regularly, at least every week.

5. If kids around me are smoking, drinking, or doing drugs:
   a. I may feel out of place, but I experience no pressure to join in.
   b. I feel very out of place and feel pressure to join, but resist.
   c. Sometimes I resist and sometimes I join in.
   d. I always smoke, drink, or do drugs with them.

6. When it comes to substances, especially alcohol and drugs, my parents:
   a. Think that doing substances can be very dangerous for adults and kids.
   b. Think that substances are okay for adults to engage in but not for kids.
   c. Don't pay much attention to drugs and alcohol either way.
   d. Think that it's perfectly fine for kids to drink and do drugs.

7. I think most kids who smoke, drink, or do drugs are:
   a. Uncool and foolish.
   b. Followers doing what kids do these days.
   c. Curious or bored.
   d. Cool and exciting.

8. The idea that illegal substances are dangerous and addictive (such that you get hooked easily and can't stop) is:
   a. Very true and something everybody should take extremely seriously.
   b. True but blown out of proportion.
   c. True for a small group of people but not for most.
   d. A myth designed to scare kids into not smoking, drinking, or doing drugs.

9. When I feel stressed out, I:
   a. Try to deal with my problems head-on.
   b. Try to distract myself with various activities, such as sports.
   c. Ignore them and hope they'll go away.
   d. I turn to cigarettes, alcohol, or drugs.

**Scoring the Quiz:** An (a) response = 1 point; (b) response = 2 points; (c) response = 3 points; and a (d) response = 4 points. When you add up your total for the quiz, if your score falls between 9 and 15, then you're On Solid Ground; between 16 and 25, then you're On Shaky Ground; and between 26 and 36, you're In Quicksand.

**On Solid Ground:** You're not at all into illegal substances and people support you in that decision. Occasionally, you may be curious, but your knowledge of the potential negative consequences of these substances keeps you on the "no" side. Also, you know how to enjoy life without illegal substances. This chapter will give you even more healthy alternatives and help fortify your approach.

**On Shaky Ground:** You're not quite sure what stance to take on illegal substances. You definitely care about your body because you've almost finished reading this entire book. This chapter will help you realistically evaluate the supposed benefits versus proven dangers of these substances. It will also strengthen your willpower and give you ideas for fun and exciting alternatives.

**In Quicksand:** Addiction is here or right around the corner. It may be tempting to deny it, but give yourself credit for answering the quiz questions honestly—you clearly want to find a way to take back control of your life. Think back to a time when you, not the substances, were in charge of your body and mind; this chapter will help you get back there, as well as help you understand how you lost control in the first place.

---

The health message that cigarette smoking is highly addictive and deadly has been sweeping the nation. In response, most Americans are reducing their smoking by quitting or never starting, except for one subgroup whose smoking is *increasing* at the fastest, steadiest rate. Do you know which group of people hasn't caught on yet? It's girls, girls your age. Why do you think?

---

## The Dilemma

Were you surprised to find out where you fall on the illegal substance scale? Where do you think Susan would fall? I'd put her in Shaky Ground territory for sure. What should we advise her to do? If my friend Ann were giving Susan guidance, she would warn, "Avoid the gathering at all costs." It's no wonder; at Ann's high school several kids died every year from alcohol poisoning, drunk driving, and the occasional drug overdose. On the other hand, if my friend Glen were giving the advice, he would say, "Go to the party; you might make some new friends." For Glen in high school, smoking pot hooked him up with a group of kids who became his pals.

My advice to Susan would be not to go to the party. Susan clearly has appropriate concerns about the dangers of smoking and drinking. Yet at the same time, it seems as though she could easily let herself be pressured into participating when she really doesn't want to. Where am I coming from? Drawing from my own experience and my work with teens, I believe that alcohol and drugs create problems and solve none: from social embarrassments to more serious health hazards, even death. It's not a morality issue of people being good or bad; it's a matter of your health and happiness. So even though I might sound like your mom or dad at times, it's because, like your parents, I care about your happiness and safety.

Have you ever thought that alcohol and drugs might help you relax in social situations or get you into the "in" crowd? Well, I've got several real life stories, including a few of my own, that might make you think otherwise.

---

The terrifying truth about cigarettes:

- Tobacco smoke contains more than 4,000 chemicals, including carbon monoxide, arsenic, and lead, and almost four dozen of the chemicals are known to cause cancer—cancer of the lungs, lips, mouth, and more.
- Because it's so poisonous, nicotine is used as the main ingredient in many products designed to kill insects.
- If a person were to inhale all at once the amount of nicotine the average pack-a-day smoker inhales in a week—400 milligrams—the person would die instantly.
- Every ten seconds, a person somewhere in the world dies from tobacco-related causes.
- Smoking is the leading cause of preventable deaths in the U.S.
- Cigarettes are the number-one cause of fires.
- Heart attacks, strokes, and kidney failure also result from smoking and can kill you.
- Smoking can cause blood clots that can lead to limbs being amputated.

## Personality Makeover

Everybody feels self-conscious during junior high and high school, even if they don't admit it. Have you ever been hanging out with a group of people, and had trouble getting up the courage to really join in the conversation? When you do bring yourself to say something, do you think, "Why did I say that?" You just can't relax, cut loose, and be comfortable being you. I know I've felt that way many times. Here's what happened to two girls when they drank alcohol with the hopes of setting themselves free:

Laura was drinking wine coolers with a bunch of friends and felt "loosened up" by the alcohol. She felt so free that she told her good friend Rose exactly what was on her mind, "You have an attitude problem. You think you're so much better than the rest of us. Get an ego check." The next day, Rose confronted Laura, "That was so messed up what you said." Laura couldn't even remember what had happened. When Rose told her, Laura denied responsibility: "Oh, that wasn't me; it was the alcohol." But Rose didn't buy that excuse and the friendship has never been the same since.

Michelle was drinking with some friends, including Max, her ex-boyfriend. She missed Max and wished that they had never broken up. Being drunk, Michelle gained the courage to share her true feelings with Max; she pulled her pants down, revealing her underwear, and said, "Max, let's get back together." The story swept through the eighth grade. Needless to say, Max and Michelle never got back together.

If you've ever embarrassed yourself or hurt people you cared about while under the influence of drugs or alcohol, there's no guarantee that the damage can be repaired, but it's worth a try. I recommend saying you're sorry, taking full responsibility for what you did, and letting them know you've learned your lesson. The maturity it takes to own up to one's mistakes and genuinely say "I'm sorry" might be enough to convince them to give you another chance.

You're just at the age now when your personality is going through a major growth spurt. The way that personalities become more dynamic is by engaging with people when you're yourself, not intoxicated. Sure, there are times when you don't like yourself and wish you were someone else. Take comfort in the fact that everyone feels that way, and then follow some suggestions for helping your personality shine forth. There's much more dynamism inside of you than you ever knew.

---

Don't be fooled:
- Light beer, beer, and wine coolers all contain plenty of alcohol.
- Even very small amounts of hard liquor—like vodka, scotch, rum, gin, and whiskey—contain a lot of alcohol.
- Just because beer and wine are advertised on TV, while hard liquor is not, doesn't mean that they're any less hazardous.
- Beer accounts for more than three-quarters of all the alcohol consumed in dangerous amounts.

---

### ACTION: The More Confident and Comfortable You

1. **Be Yourself.** By being yourself, you attract people who adore you for who you are. This is what I did in high school; even though it meant riding out some awkward times, it paid off big time with friendships that I still have today.
2. **Have a Base Buddy.** Find at least one friend who makes you feel cherished. Whenever you're someplace, whether at a party or hanging out with kids after school, and you feel like you want a personality makeover, check in with your base buddy as a reminder that you're great just the way you are.

3. **Find an Extracurricular Home.** Whether it's a sports team, a drama club, or a school orchestra, find a group of kids who are doing what you like to do. There's nothing like a common interest to bring down the awkwardness barriers. (See the website for some ideas.)

4. **Ask Questions.** Wondering what to say to somebody new? Most people love to answer questions about themselves. And if they have real friend potential, they'll ask you questions in return.

5. **Build Body Comfort.** Sometimes it's simply not knowing what to do with your arms and legs that distracts you from enjoying yourself: limbs crossed, uncrossed, dangling, fidgeting—you know what I mean. Take a martial arts, yoga, or dance class to help you feel more relaxed. My favorite way to loosen up at parties has always been to dance. But if dancing makes you more self-conscious, then practice at home, alone or with friends; no fancy moves required—just listen to the beat and have fun!

---

Warning: Some inhalants can kill you within minutes by giving you a heart attack. Inhalants have also killed teens by causing car crashes due to blurred vision, sleepiness, and nausea. What is an inhalant? Any substance that emits fumes or comes in an aerosol form; these include nitrous oxide (laughing gas), amyl nitrite ("poppers" or "snappers"), butyl nitrite ("rush" or "bolt"), spray paint, gasoline, paint thinner, and glue.

---

## From Fitting In to Giving In

Have you ever been with a bunch of people and wanted to be part of their crowd, be ONE of THEM? The desire to be close to people is a healthy one. However, the situation can get tricky when the desire to belong ends up making you do things you normally wouldn't do.

My freshman year of college, a bunch of older guys who usually didn't pay much attention to me invited me out to drink with them. They were drinking shots of tequila, with beer to chase it down, so I was too. I remember thinking, "They must think I'm so cool for keeping up with them," when all of a sudden the liquor hit me all at once and I became violently ill. I made it to the bathroom just in time to vomit somewhere close to the toilet. My insides just kept coming up and out, up and out. I was totally alone and terrified. Eventually, the vomiting subsided and my close friends Sandra and John appeared out of nowhere; the drinking guys had called them to come take me home. Back home in bed, I felt ill, confused, and more embarrassed than I had ever been. By wanting to fit in, I ended up standing out in ways I never ever wanted to.

> Girls are more susceptible to alcohol's effects due to their smaller size, lower percentage of water in their bodies, and a fact that few people know—a body enzyme that helps metabolize alcohol is less active in females than in males.

I'm happy to say that I have never had nearly that much to drink again. The experience also helped me see clearly with whom I wanted to be friends and whom I didn't. I felt insecure and uncomfortable with the older guys to begin with, which is why I drank. True friendships have breathing room for individuality and space for you to test out and assert who you are. Engaging in drug and alcohol use provides an artificial sense of belonging. What kind of real friend would drop you if you decided not to smoke?

Sometimes pressure to use these substances is as direct as somebody saying, "Hey, smoke this." But more often the pressure is indirect; you're surrounded by people smoking or drinking and you want to fit in. I never lost a friend by politely turning down substances. But I did find that I tended to hang out more with people who did things that made me say, "Yes, thanks." The choice is yours, and here are a few tips for how to quietly stand your ground.

> Forty percent of teens *strongly* believe that "kids who are really cool don't use drugs." Only eight percent agreed with the statement that "pot smokers are popular."

### ACTION: Fight the Pressure

1. **Redirection.** If your friends always drink or do drugs when you're together, try motivating them to do a new activity, such as roller-blading or ice skating, that requires sobriety if they plan to stand up for any length of time.

2. **Substance Abusers Are in the Minority.** Remind yourself that for every kid who is using, there are at least two to three kids who aren't. If you want to find fun, sober, nonsmokers to hang with, there are plenty of kids to choose from; just look around your school and community.

> Research found that kids overestimate how many of their friends and classmates smoke, drink, or have tried drugs. Since this misperception can be a strong motivator to engage in taking these substances, here are a few recent statistics to provide the real story:
>
> Four out of five adolescents do *not* do drugs.
>
> Two out of three teens do *not* smoke.
>
> Three out of four eighth graders have never been drunk.

3. **Brainstorm and Role-Play.** Think of all the different pressure situations you might find yourself in and write down how you would deal with them. Ask a good friend to do the same and then role-play the scenes and your responses.

4. **"No, thanks" or "Maybe later."** If you find yourself in a bind, try saying what always worked for me, "No, thanks" in a confident yet non-judgmental tone. Or try saying, "Maybe later"; by the time later rolls around, everybody is too wasted to notice that you never joined in.

5. **Hold Off.** If you find yourself being tempted, tell yourself, "I'll say 'No, thanks' and when I'm away from the pressure, I'll think out my position. If I choose to try it, there will always be other opportunities."

6. **Be Elsewhere.** The best way to refuse is by planning to hang out where drugs and alcohol aren't.

7. **If You've Tried an Illegal Substance.** If you gave into peer pressure and tried smoking or drinking, don't be hard on yourself; just use the experience to tell people, "I tried ____ and it made me nauseated and gave me a really bad headache. I think I'll skip it." And don't let yourself develop amnesia. If you liked the experience and are considering doing more, answer these questions honestly: Am I in control and can I trust the people around me?

8. **Get Assistance.** If you are experiencing unrelenting pressure to engage in substance abuse or even to help sell drugs, consult an adult in your life or community on how to handle the situation. Consider joining an after-school program or sport.

---

Don't be fooled:
- Filtered cigarettes are just as hazardous to your health as regular cigarettes.
- Lower-nicotine cigarettes can be equally dangerous because the smoker usually inhales more and smokes more often.
- Smokeless tobacco that you snuff or chew still causes cancer.

## Who's the Boss Here?

You do what you're supposed to do: go to school, eat the foods served to you, do your homework (well, most of the time), and keep your room relatively neat (well, at least you don't keep old candy bars lying around). Sometimes you feel like everybody else is dictating your life, saying, "Do this, don't do that." You're wondering where YOU come into the equation; when do you get a say in your own life?

Wishing to assert your individuality is something I applaud wholeheartedly. The question is: What's the best way to go about it? Most likely your parents have cautioned you against cigarettes, alcohol, and drugs—forbidden substances equal instant rebellion. But an instant of rebellion can lead to many more rules and restrictions. Here's one of the milder stories I've collected:

Fourteen-year-old Jennie was hanging out with friends and got so drunk and sick that she couldn't move without becoming overwhelmingly nauseated. When she wasn't home by 2:30 A.M., her parents were worried sick and frantically called the parents of all Jennie's friends trying to locate her. Her parents were getting ready to call the police, when Jennie finally staggered in the door at 4:00 A.M. Her parents hugged and kissed her with relief; they were upset that she didn't call, when for all they knew she had been killed in a drunk driving accident. Wanting to keep their daughter safe from harm, they took away her house key privileges and instituted a strict curfew of midnight—limitations they had never even considered establishing before.

If it's the fact that your parents are forbidding you to smoke or drink that makes you want to do these activities all the more, then find your own reasons for wanting to abstain. Maybe they focus on the dangers, but for you the potential social embarrassment could be the main turn-off. Hurting yourself to stand up to your parents only gets them breathing down your neck more and is much more harmful to your life than to theirs. I felt fortunate growing up because I had an unspoken agreement with my parents; they trusted me to make sound judgments when it came to substance abuse and sex, and in return for being responsible, they gave me a ton of freedom.

Here are some fun, safe ways to assert your independence.

---

Thinking of trying cigarettes? If you do, odds are you will be stuck smoking for the rest of your life:

- Nicotine is at least as addictive as cocaine or heroin and just as difficult to stop using.
- Two-thirds of adolescents who smoke say they wish they had never started and want to quit.
- Ninety-two percent of teens who smoke said that they wouldn't be smoking a year later, but only 1.5 percent of these kids managed to quit.
- Approximately 90 percent of all tobacco users start before age 18.

---

### ACTION: Hear You Roar

True rebellion shows signs of creativity.

1. **Take Steps Toward Independence.** Start your own business, redecorate your room, get involved in the planning of the family vacation.
2. **Be the Voice of Your Generation.** Make your opinions heard. You've got a lot to say that the world needs to hear. Find a way to speak out—whether it's through making a video, joining a youth group, painting, writing songs, or creating sculptures. (See the website for ways to explore your potential and have a voice.)
3. **Push Limits Within Your Area of Interest.** Whether it be computers, science, music, art, or writ-

ing, take a field somewhere it's never been before. Create art to be reckoned with. Did you know that kids who win the Westinghouse Science Talent Search have often made unique contributions to the field of science?

4. **Want to Dip into the "Forbidden"?** Meet secretly in the girls' bathroom to hold a book or magazine club in which you all read the same material and discuss what you liked and what you thought was bogus.

5. **Take Advantage of Your Kid Status.** As a girl, I enjoyed the fact that homework and piano practice were my only responsibilities. I loved having my birthday be a very special day and being cared for when I was sick. What do you like about being a kid? Enjoy the perks that come with youth.

---

Don't smoke hemp, the plant that marijuana is made from, but why not wear it or write on it? For thousands of years, the fiber from the hemp plant has been used to make clothing, rope, and paper. The first drafts of the American Declaration of Independence were written on hemp paper and Betsy Ross sewed the American flag using hemp.

---

## The High Life

Ever felt that life was a bit dull? The same school, same teachers, same friends, and of course, the same parents and house to go home to. According to everybody else, you've got a great life, but according to you, your life is lame. Anything exciting going on in your town, like a great band playing or a hip dance scene, seems to require that you're 21. You feel stuck in Dullsville, USA.

Then you hear kids at school bragging about what an amazing time they had over the weekend getting "smashed" and "wasted," and you think, "Now there's some excitement waiting to happen." And you're tempted to try to join them next weekend or to get your friends to try drinking with you. But what you don't know is the real story behind their weekend party. The words "smashed" and "wasted" should give you a clue. In all likelihood, at least one person was throwing up in the bathroom, another was passed out on the couch, and everybody was too hungover the next day to go inline skating or study for the big algebra exam. Plus, they probably can hardly remember what happened since heavy alcohol and drug use dulls the memory or can even cause blackouts.

> Did you know that sexual activities are not the only way that the deadly AIDS virus is spread? The virus lives in blood. That's why doctors and nurses make sure to use fresh, clean needles on patients and why intravenous (I.V.) drug users who inject the illegal substances are strongly advised not to share needles.

My college roommate used to brag all the time about the amazing experiences she had while doing this and that drug. I always wondered whether or not I was missing out on something great. But then one time she and I snuck into a political fund-raising party for a presidential candidate; it was much more boring than we expected. The next week, I overheard her telling somebody what an exciting time we had had at the fund-raiser. So whenever you hear people boasting about how much fun they had when they were wasted, think of my ex-roommate and tell yourself that they're probably not telling you the real story.

So now you're thinking, "Great, if smoking and drinking won't do it, I'm still stuck in the doldrums—get me out!" You, my dear, have the power to pull yourself out on your own. You don't need something or someone to sweep you away. When my friends and I talk about the most exciting times of our lives, these were not times that we were in-toxicated—instead it was meeting somebody new or special, exploring a place or an art or a sport we'd never done before. Here are some ideas to spark your own sense of adventure.

---

Which type of companies spend the most money on advertising? The tobacco and alcohol companies, and it's no wonder! With 1,200 adult smokers dying each day, the tobacco industry has to recruit new smokers to stay in business. Considering the number of deadly drunk driving accidents and the physical damage alcohol causes, we could say something similar about the alcohol industry.

---

### ACTION: Adding Spice to Your Life—From Salt to Paprika

1. **Get Out There.** Photograph your town. Make a new friend who is from another country by being a pen or E-mail pal (who knows, maybe you'll be able to visit someday). Go horseback riding, surfing, swimming, camping, mountain biking, or on a safari at a big zoo. Be a tourist in your own city with the help of a guidebook or even a guided tour.
2. **Spend an Afternoon in a Bookstore.** Read new books and magazines, and do research for future missions. Use travel guides, crafts books, and publishing guides to find out to which magazines you can send your poetry and stories.
3. **Join Others in Their Adventures.** Ask a sister, brother, or friend what their favorite exciting yet safe activities are and ask if you can come along on the next journey.
4. **Try Something You've Never Done Before.** Just the newness makes it exciting.
5. **Make Your Own Adventure.** If there are any you've discovered and loved, send your suggestions my way and I'll post them on the website for other girls to try.

What drug is on the rise among teens? Ecstasy (or "X").
This drug is often used by teens to fuel all night dance
sessions. Don't be fooled by tablets in the shape of fun and
innocent-looking dinosaurs or Buddhas; this drug is
dangerous. It can lead to fainting, muscle cramps, panic
attacks, blurred vision, paranoia, nausea, memory loss, and
more.

## No Way Out

Let's face it, life in teenland is not all fun and games. There
are pressures to succeed in school, please your parents, and
be popular, not to mention coping with stressful family and
friend situations. Sometimes you want to cry out, "I'm not
a kid anymore—look at all I have to deal with! Leave me
alone!"

Drugs and alcohol can become tempting during stressful
times. A guy I knew in high school, Larry, started stressing
out majorly when his parents started fighting all the time
and threatening each other with divorce. Then his parents
split up and each started pressuring him to come live with
them. Larry didn't know what to do, so he started drinking
and drugging. Pretty soon he was cutting classes, and pretty
soon his grades dropped to near failing. His old friends
stopped hanging out with him, while his new ones were
always trying to hit him up for money for drugs. On top
of all that, his parents said that until Larry's grades came
back up, he couldn't play in his band—Larry's one positive
stress releaser.

Alcohol acts as a depressant on your brain and nervous
system—tears in the beer.

By turning to drugs and alcohol, Larry made his life
harder, rather than easier. As a girl, I had worries, but I

also had a certain philosophy that always got me through the rough spots; if you try to ignore or cover over pain, you'll only end up feeling worse in the end. But if you tackle problems, they can only get better.

You might be thinking, "Well, I can see that with drugs and alcohol, but how about smoking; aren't cigarettes supposed to make you more relaxed?" A recent study found that when smokers are not smoking, they experience *more* stress than nonsmokers do. The brains of smokers come to depend on the presence of nicotine to feel "normal." When the nicotine isn't coursing through smokers' bloodstreams, they feel irritable and stressed out.

---

Smokers suffer from 65 percent more colds, 167 percent more irritations of the throat and nose, and are 300 percent more likely to develop chronic coughs than nonsmokers.

---

You'll be happy to know that nature has given each of us our own healthy de-stressing, happiness drug—**endorphins**: that natural high that your sports groove releases. So if life is getting you down, instead of saying to yourself, "I can't handle this—I give up," grab your athletic wear and try these actions:

### . ACTION: De-Stressing the Healthy Way
1. **Get Your Sports Groove On.** Exercise to release your natural happiness substance or take a yoga class to relax. If you're still feeling blue, go on to step #2.
2. **Try the Thought Tracer Technique.** This strategy, described on page 175, will help you determine the main trouble that's bringing you down and making you anxious.
3. **Let It Out.** Write in your journal, talk to a parent or another adult, or speak with a friend.
4. **Get Practical Assistance.** If you're anxious about

schoolwork, ask a parent, friend, teacher, or tutor for assistance.
5. **Get Professional Help.** If the troubles in your life feel overwhelming, see Chapter 10 on Seeking Help.

---

Just hanging out on a regular basis with smokers in the girls' bathroom could give you more colds, allergies, or asthma. Of the 4,000 chemicals contained in secondhand smoke, 60 were found to be cancer-causing. People can develop lung cancer and die from secondhand smoke.

---

## Just Wondering ...

Everybody thinks at some point, "Hmmm ... I wonder what it would feel like to be drunk, or high, or smoke a cigarette? Why doesn't anyone trust me to be able to handle myself? A drink or two certainly isn't going to kill me." The problem is that under certain circumstances, it might. I don't mean to be alarmist, but I learned this lesson the hard way; I'm hoping that you can learn from my mistakes.

When I was 16, I went to a party of college students on the Jersey shore—a house full of music and cute guys, what could be better? Everybody was drinking and I'd never gotten drunk before, so I thought, "Why not now? If I make a fool of myself, I'll never see these people again anyway." So I drank a few beers and got drunk, but to be honest, I was feeling kind of bored because I didn't know anybody except for my friend who was busy flirting with a guy. So when a couple of guys invited me to go for a ride in their new convertible, I jumped at the chance.

We got in the car and sped off, really fast, way faster than all the cars we passed and almost hit. While taking me on the terror ride of my life, these guys were laughing. Being drunk, they actually thought the near-death experience was fun. My requests that they please slow down were ignored; I fastened my seat belt, held on, and prayed. Fortunately, we returned to the party relatively quickly, but in my terror, it seemed like an eternity.

When I got out of the car, I was shaking from fright, and one of the guys reached out to me. I thought he was trying to comfort me; no—he was making a sexual pass. Since I had been drunk and gone along for the ride, he was hoping I'd go along for another kind of ride. I was too drunk and scared to know what to do. Fortunately, the other guy said, "Save it for later," giving me enough time to dash into the house, find my friend, and not leave her side again.

---

What is the leading killer of young Americans ages 15 to 24? Alcohol-related car crashes:

- Even just a small amount of alcohol or drugs can severely impair the coordination and judgment required for safe driving.
- Nothing can speed up the rate at which somebody sobers up—not a cold shower, not fresh air, not a cup of coffee—nothing. In fact, coffee may *increase* the negative effects of alcohol, even if the person "feels" more alert.
- Despite these dangerous facts, over a third of high school students said they had ridden with a driver who had been drinking alcohol.
- Don't get in the car—this could save your life. There's always a safer way to get where you need to go; call a friend or parents, or just stay put for a while. If you're worried about what parents will say, let them know that you feel you made a mistake and you're trying to do the responsible thing right now—come pick me up, please!

---

I could very easily have been killed in that car ride or even raped by one or both of the guys. The sober me would have known better than to have ever gotten into that car in the first place. But the drunk me wanted to go along for the ride. Alcohol and drugs take away our natural instincts that we depend on to sense danger and keep ourselves safe from harm. I was lucky to have survived, but thousands of kids every year aren't as lucky. The high statistics on drunk driving accidents don't even include the kids who die in other types of accidents while inebriated. I knew a boy in high school who was high on drugs and was killed by a car when he crossed the road. I knew another boy who went swimming in a reservoir while drunk and drowned.

The impaired judgment that comes with having a couple of drinks can also lead to your having two more drinks, then two more, and so on. Too much alcohol in a small period of time can lead to alcohol poisoning which can kill. With alcohol poisoning, you don't know how much is going to be deadly until it's too late. With drugs, it's impossible to know exactly what you're dealing with each time. Drugs are unregulated because they're illegal. Essentially the potency and toxicity are a mystery, and most illegal drugs are laced with other harmful or even deadly chemicals. This is why drug overdoses happen fairly often.

> People who pass out from consuming too much alcohol can easily throw up while sleeping, choke on their own vomit, and even *die*. If you're with someone who passes out from too much drinking, roll her onto her side into the "fetal position" and call 911.

Trying alcohol or drugs once or twice typically can lead to doing more and more—that's also what makes them so dangerous. It's like when you open a bag of potato chips or cookies and say, "I'll just have one," and of course you don't—how can you resist? It's not that you don't have willpower; it's that you're human. You're in an age group that's extra vulnerable; the large majority of substance addiction begins during the preteen and teen years. Your growing and developing body is extra-sensitive. Your personality is finding itself, so it too is tender. While adults are vulnerable to addiction, kids are even more so.

You may be thinking, "But who really *never* tries even one cigarette?" I've met plenty of people who haven't, and now you can say you definitely know at least one person who hasn't—me. I've never had even a puff. I'm not interested and never will be. There's another substance I've mentioned that I've never had a puff of either—marijuana. There have been plenty of opportunities for me to smoke pot, but I didn't want to. Sure, I was curious, but only mildly so. For me, these substances have never seemed all that appealing, and the risks involved make them just not worth a try.

Don't get me wrong, I have a healthy curiosity and act on it in many different ways, including visiting countries all over the world, trying raw oysters and snails at restaurants, and acting as mother to a baby monkey for a week. I bet that the number of things you're curious about could fill this book. Curiosity is a great thing; it's what keeps the body of scientific knowledge growing and makes people get to know each other. So for right now, why not choose to explore your healthier curiosities? You don't have to make decisions right now for the rest of your life, just for what's better for you during the teen years. By the time you're in your twenties, you might just have found more exciting things to explore—like foreign countries or romance. In the meantime . . .

---

Drinking alcohol greatly increases the odds that you'll be involved in a violent crime, either as the victim or the perpetrator:

> A study conducted at American colleges found that alcohol was involved in 90 percent of rapes, 95 percent of violent crimes, and 66 percent of student suicides.
>
> Much more than half of state prisoners convicted of violent crimes had used alcohol just before the offense.

### *ACTION: A Healthy Curiosity*

1. **Take Up an Art Form from Another Culture.**
   Study a dance, music, painting, or martial art form
   that comes from another part of the world.
2. **Time Travel.** Learn how people lived many decades
   or centuries ago by going to museums or reading fic-
   tion that takes place in other times.
3. **Explore and Learn.** Read books and watch docu-
   mentaries that make your head spin—books about
   people who climbed the world's highest mountain or
   films about how animals survive in the desert. Then
   go visit a mountain or a desert.
4. **Meet People from Other Cultures.** Get to know
   people from other parts of the U.S. and from other
   countries by attending their local holiday festivals or
   taking special dance, music or martial arts classes.
5. **Travel.** Encourage your family to take a trip somewhere you have never been.

---

Here's the straight dope on marijuana:
  • Marijuana is much stronger today than it was back in
    the 1960s, or even a decade ago.
  • Marijuana has just as many, if not more, cancer-causing
    agents than do cigarettes. (Smoking five joints per week
    may expose a person to as much of a cancer risk as
    smoking a full pack of cigarettes each day.)

---

## One Last Reason . . .

Looking for an energy lift? Sure, a drink or a cigarette or
a drug might give you a brief boost, but soon enough, it
will leave you feeling worse than before you used the substance, plus you'll have de-energizing side effects, such as

headaches and nausea. Your body has you covered with your own natural energizing substance—**adrenaline**—which kicks in when you need it; that's how I pulled through all-night paper-writing sessions in college. This section doesn't need an action to follow because this entire book is a guide on how to eat, exercise, and sleep well so that you'll have all the energy you need and then some.

---

The down phase of illegal substance use lasts much longer than the up phase. There's no cure for alcohol's hangover, which includes headaches, upset stomach, shakiness, and can last one to two days. Here's something most people don't know: Pot stays in your system for up to seven days, decreasing your memory and coordination for at least three days, if not more.

---

## What Puts You at Risk for Substance Abuse?

Have you ever wondered why it is that some kids resist trying alcohol, tobacco, and drugs, while others don't? And why some kids become addicted while some don't? Different kids have different risk and protective factors. In fact, most of the factors I discussed in the eating disorder chapter apply here. The main difference lies in the behavior of family and friends. In the last chapter, the troubled behavior of loved ones revolved around food, such as dieting; here it centers on drugs and alcohol.

---

In the United States, one out of ten adults suffers from alcoholism. This means that millions of kids have parents who are alcoholics or know friends whose parents are.

If you have a parent who is addicted to alcohol or drugs, it can be extremely difficult and scary to see your parent so out of control. Parents who are intoxicated typically become neglectful, verbally abusive with undeserved criticism, and may even be physically or sexually abusive. Because addiction can be (but isn't always) passed down from parents to their kids, you are at risk for substance abuse big-time. Genetics certainly play a large role; in addition, parents serve as role models, for better or for worse. Don't panic, just play it safe and follow the 100 percent fail-proof way of protecting yourself: Avoid alcohol or drugs *completely*, do not even take a single puff, sip, or pill.

---

One-third of Americans report that they drink no alcohol at all. Overall, alcohol use has been on the decline among adults. Why do you think this is? Experts attribute part of the decline to the increasing emphasis on being healthy and fit.

---

If, however, you have parents who don't engage in substance abuse and do talk about the harm substances inflict, then you'll be much less likely to give into substances yourself. So how do you protect yourself when parents aren't protecting themselves? Read on.

### ACTION: What to Do If Parents Are Abusing

1. **Take Care of Yourself.** Remember that just because a parent is unable to be a good role model, this doesn't mean that you can't do right for yourself.
2. **Be Extra Cautious.** Be aware that you're very vulnerable to becoming addicted and that abstaining is by far the safest approach you can take.
3. **You Cannot Be the Rescuer.** Convince yourself of

the truth—the truth being that your parents' struggles are neither your fault nor your responsibility. You cannot rescue them or be their cover-up accomplice; she or he needs help from professionals.

4. **Get Support.** Because living with an addicted parent is so difficult, there are groups especially for you to get support; these include Alateen, Al-Anon and NA (Narcotics Anonymous). (See resource listings at end of this chapter.) Helping yourself is the best way for you to help your parents.

5. **Be Safe.** If your parent is sexually or physically abusing you, go directly to page 244 and read the chapter on getting professional help.

6. **Worried About a Friend?** If you're concerned about a friend who's abusing, then get a helpful adult involved, but remember—your friend won't change until she's ready.

7. **Have a Life.** Another risk factor for substance abuse is having few interests or activities, so get out there and find your sports groove and other passions that make you tick.

---

Since most addiction to tobacco, alcohol, and drugs takes hold during the teen years, the U.S. government is trying to prevent drug use among kids by:

- Creating legal age limits for purchasing and using alcohol and cigarettes
- Establishing drug-free school zones, so that anyone caught with drugs within 1,000 feet of school property receives severe legal penalties. (Did you ever notice a sign near your school?)
- Cracking down on drunk driving by making punishment more severe (It works to prevent deaths!)

And more. What do you think of these strategies? What type of prevention program would you put into action?

> The government in Quebec, Canada, is planning to deter
> smoking by decorating cigarette packages with full-color
> photos of cancerous lips and lungs: lungs that are
> blackened, shriveled, and scarred.

## Getting Help

If you're already finding that a substance has gotten hold
of you, don't panic. There are many services and organizations out there designed to help you break your addiction
or to quit before the addiction kicks in. You can start by
trying to quit on your own cold-turkey, but be prepared for
withdrawal symptoms and a battle. For smoking, there are
nicotine replacement products, like gums, patches, and pre-
scription drugs as well as hypnosis or acupuncture. For
drugs and alcohol, there are therapists, hospital clinics, and
community support groups, like Alcoholics Anonymous
(AA), Narcotics Anonymous (NA), and Rational Recovery
(RR) groups. Congratulate yourself for admitting that you
need help and then go get it. The next chapter is devoted
to getting you the help you need, so use the resources listed
in this chapter and keep on reading.

## The Benefits of Abstaining

The benefits of not engaging in substance abuse are abun-
dant. To name a few: You feel happier, have more money
in your pocket, handle stress better, have more satisfying
friendships, can appreciate your own natural highs, and are
free to do what you want, not what a substance wants you
to do. That's the whole point of this book—to help you
take charge of your body and mind in a healthy way. I
hope this chapter has helped you sort out some of your

feelings about tobacco, alcohol, and drugs and given you appealing alternatives to consider.

If you're currently struggling with your own or a parent's substance abuse, or if at any point while reading the chapters in this book, you thought, "I wish I had someone to talk to about this," then make sure to read the next chapter on getting help. Even if there's nothing troubling you right now, why not check out the short chapter to keep the information on file for future reference? Also, don't forget to say good-bye—the very last chapter is my chance to say good-bye to you.

---

How much do you think a typical pack-a-day smoker spends on cigarettes in five years? Approximately $8,700.

---

## Check Out These Resources

### Phone Numbers and Websites

Drug Help (For alcohol or drugs)
1 (800) 378-4435 (24-hours: Counseling, answers to questions, and referrals for counselors near you.)
*www.drughelp.org*

Alcohol and Drug Referral Line
1 (800) 821-4357 (24-hours: Referrals to a local counselor for any issues concerning alcohol or drug use.)

Al-Anon and Alateen (Support for kids whose parents abuse alcohol or drugs)
(888) 4-AL-ANON or 1 (800) 344-2666 (Regular weekday hours: For Al-Anon/Alateen meeting referrals, and further information.)
Web sites: *http://www.alateen.org* or *http://www.al-anon.alateen.org/*

Alcoholics Anonymous (AA) and Narcotics Anonymous (NA)

Look in your local phone book or call directory assistance for the branch nearest you.

(212) 647-1680 (24-hours, but *not* toll-free: A recovering alcoholic is there to speak with you.)

Website: *http://www.alcoholics-anonymous.org*

American Cancer Society Smoker Quitline

1 (800) 227-2345 (24-hours: Referrals to local quitting programs and information on smoking's dangers and how to quit.)

Web sites: *http://www.cancer.org*

General crisis counseling: Kid Save Hotline: 1 (800) 543-7283 or National Runaway Switchboard: 1 (800) 621-4000.

*http://stopdrugs.org/*: Deals with both prevention and treatment of drug-related problems.

*http://www.alcoholismhelp.com*: Provides help with alcoholism.

*zaphealth.com*: This site provides information for teens on sex, drugs, alcohol, mental health, family problems, skin problems, weight issues, and sports injuries. You can ask an expert for advice.

## Books

Cheney, Glenn A. *Drugs, Teens, and Recovery: Real-Life Stories of Trying to Stay Clean*. Springfield, New Jersey: Enslow Publishers, 1993.

Folkers, Gladys, and Jeanne Engelman. *Taking Charge of My Mind and Body: A Girl's Guide to Outsmarting Al-*

cohol, Drugs, Smoking, and Eating Problems*. Minneapolis: Free Spirit Publishing, 1997.

McMillan, Daniel. *Teen Smoking: Understanding the Risk (Issues in Focus)*. Springfield, New Jersey: Enslow Publishers, Inc., 1998.

Ryan, Elizabeth. *Straight Talk about Drugs and Alcohol*. New York: Facts on File, 1995.

Ryerson, Eric. *When Your Parent Drinks Too Much: A Book for Teenagers*. New York: Facts on File, 1985.

Scoppettone, Sandra, and David Rogers. *The Late Great Me*. New York: Dramatic Publishing Company, 1977.

# TEN

# Take Good Care of Yourself— Seeking Help

While reading in this book about the stresses girls can feel, were there any moments when you thought, "I'd like to talk with somebody about what's on my mind"? If so, did the thought of meeting with a counselor seem comforting and yet scary all at once? That's understandable; something unfamiliar is often a little scary, especially when it involves sharing your secret thoughts with a stranger. In this chapter I'll try to make the unfamiliar more familiar by discussing what happens when you call a hotline number or visit a counselor. Even if you're feeling pretty good about your life right now, why not read the chapter and keep the information filed away for the future? You never know when the urge to see a counselor might hit.

## No Trouble Is Too Big or Too Small

When you're feeling sad or angry, my guess is that sometimes you're also feeling alone and hopeless, as if nothing could make the problem better. I want to assure you that no matter how much you may think that nobody cares about how you're feeling—there are plenty of people who do. No matter how hopeless your problem may seem—there's plenty of hope. Maybe you feel that what's troubling you is small in comparison to other people's troubles; I'm here to tell you that whatever it is that's getting you down, it's important and worthy of attention. So whatever your concerns, no matter how overwhelmingly difficult or how seemingly small, there are people waiting by phones and sitting in offices wanting to help you.

When I worked as a high school counselor in Berkeley, California, girls came to me looking for help with a whole range of concerns. One girl talked about how her mom was high on drugs all the time, leaving her to care for herself and her younger brother. Another girl spoke about being nervous that she and her boyfriend were considering having sex. Another girl came to see me because she was confused about puberty and all the changes that were happening to her body. There are many different things that might be bringing you down, and therapy can help with any problem. There's no problem that you should feel stupid or embarrassed to share.

I know for certain that therapy can help you feel less alone and more in charge of your life: less sad and anxious, more hopeful and happy. How can I be so sure? Well, not only have I counseled girls, but I've gone to a counselor myself; I can tell you firsthand that it made me feel much better.

---

There are support groups for every type of problem you can imagine. For example, there are groups for people whose beloved pets have died, people who are trying to quit smoking, or who procrastinate (i.e., put things off).

---

## Seeking Help Shows Strength

You may feel like asking for help is a sign of weakness, as if you're saying to the world, "I can't handle this on my own." In reality, the exact opposite is true; seeking assistance is a definite sign of strength. It means that you have the maturity to recognize when you need some support and have the courage to reach out and get it. By asking for help, you're taking control of the situation. You're saying, "I'm unhappy; please work with me to help make these bad feelings go away."

Sometimes girls worry that if they seek counseling, other people will think they're crazy. The adults and kids who might actually think this are those very same people who don't understand what therapy is all about. But now you know more about therapy than they do, as well as about the strength it takes to seek assistance.

---

An intense fear of something specific is a phobia. The most common is the fear of heights—acrophobia. You've probably heard of claustrophobia: the fear of being in an enclosed place. But I bet you've never heard of archibutyrophobia: the fear of peanut butter sticking to the roof of your mouth.

---

## What Counseling Is All About

You're probably wondering how this partnership works between a counselor and you. A counselor wants to listen to what's on your mind, hear what makes you sad, mad, and worried. She or he might ask you questions in order to gain a better understanding of how you're feeling and what's going on in your life. Sometimes you may go in with a clear understanding of what's troubling you, and other times it may be more of a mystery that s/he helps you solve.

In some instances, just knowing that somebody hears and understands you is enough to greatly lessen the pain you're feeling. Remember my gay friend Tony who went to see his high school guidance counselor? For him, just hearing that the feelings he was experiencing were normal was enough to ease his mind.

Many times, feeling understood helps a lot, but there's also an issue that needs problem-solving action. In that case, the counselor and you will work together on devising positive strategies, such as how to tell your mom that you feel hurt when she criticizes you, or how to let a boyfriend know that you're not ready for sex. In between counseling sessions, you can try out the strategies in your real life. When you see your therapist again, you can talk about how the plan worked and how you're feeling about it. You continue to problem-solve together until you can understand and cope with the issues in your life, and feel happy and comfortable again.

A counselor is a great partner when trying to resolve difficult situations and strong emotions; she draws not only from her professional training, but also from her experience working with other girls, some of whom have probably been in similar situations.

---

Everybody dreams, but some people remember their dreams more easily than others do. If you remember your dreams, try writing them down in a journal and thinking about their personal meaning. Many therapists believe that interpreting your dreams is a helpful way of understanding what's troubling you.

---

## Not All Therapy Is Exactly the Same

Maybe you've tried seeing a counselor before but felt that she didn't understand where you were coming from. It's important to remember that different therapists have different styles, just like different people have different personalities. Some counselors' styles might match your personality better than others, so don't give up looking until you find one you like and can talk to.

So far I've talked about seeing a counselor on your own, but you could also see a therapist with your family or with a group of girls who are struggling with similar issues. A family therapist can help resolve problems between family members and make things better at home. In group therapy, a counselor assists the girls in expressing their emotions and problem-solving together.

> There are even multifamily groups in which several different families meet together with one or two therapists.

## Whom To Talk To

Talking about what's on your mind may seem awkward, embarrassing, or scary at first, but once you start sharing your feelings, it becomes easier and easier, until it feels downright natural. Remember, professional counselors know that being a kid isn't easy and they've heard girls talk about all sorts of problems, almost anything you can think of. There are so many different ways to go about seeking help that you're guaranteed to find it. If one means doesn't work out, then try another.

**AN ADULT YOU KNOW AND TRUST:** Because the first time you share your troubles with somebody is often the hardest, some girls find it easier to start by speaking with an adult whom they already know and trust: a parent, aunt or uncle, teacher, religious leader (e.g., your priest or rabbi), doctor, or perhaps a coach. Sometimes, just telling your worries to a sympathetic ear can be enough to help you feel more secure and relaxed. But, most often, speaking with someone you know is the first step. The second step is enlisting the adult as an ally in your search for a counselor who can help you feel in charge of your life.

Why can't an adult who's already in your life be your counselor? Adults you're close to aren't trained in therapy, plus they have blind spots when it comes to how they see you—they're too close to you to get any perspective on your troubles. For example, your mother may see your sister as faultless and not understand why you and she are fighting so much. Their blind spots might also lead to their not taking your concerns seriously enough. Maybe your mom can't see how much pain you're in because she has struggled with the same problem herself, or maybe your dad's love for you makes it too upsetting for him to open his eyes to your distress. But this doesn't mean that your problem isn't important or that they don't care about you. Here's how to find a professional who can help.

**SCHOOL COUNSELOR:** While some girls prefer to start by speaking with an adult they know, others feel more comfortable talking with somebody they don't know—a professional. A great place to start is by seeking advice from your school counselor. Most schools have a psychological counselor whose sole job is to help students who are struggling with personal issues. The amazing thing about school counselors is that they are right there in your school, free of charge, and are familiar with what life is like in your school and community. To meet with your school counselor, you talk with a teacher or school nurse about making an appointment, or go directly to the counselor's office. If she's busy seeing another student, you can wait until he/she is done.

**COMMUNITY COUNSELOR:** If your school doesn't have a counselor or you'd feel more comfortable seeking help outside of your school, don't worry; there are many different free resources in your community for you to choose from. Services are set up in community centers, hospitals, and clinics specifically to help kids who have troubles on their minds. Want to know how to find them? You can start by looking in your White Pages telephone book in the county or state government pages (they're marked in blue). Look under "Health and Hospitals," "Mental Health," and "Children." These offices, however, are often closed evenings and weekends. You can also contact the organizations and 24-hour hotlines that I list at the end of chapters; the people there can answer your questions and refer you to a free community counselor near you. Once you have a phone number for a clinic, call up and make an appointment.

> Concerned about whether or not you'll be able to find a counselor? With approximately half a million therapists in the United States, odds are good that there's a counselor near you.

**HOTLINE:** You might feel more comfortable opening up to somebody over the telephone whom you don't know. The wonderful thing about a hotline number is that specially trained counselors are waiting by the phone just for your call. Most often, the phone lines are staffed round the clock, which is a tremendous help because the blues can hit hard in the middle of the night when you might be feeling extremely lonely. You can call to talk about a specific issue, to ask a question, or just because you're feeling down and can't quite pinpoint what has you so troubled. You don't have to worry about anybody in your house finding out you called; the call is free, so it doesn't appear on your parents' phone bill. You can call one of the hotlines listed in this book for specific issues or call the general hotline numbers provided.

**911:** I'm sure you're familiar with this free-of-charge phone number—it gives you a direct line to the police department. When and why would you call them? If you're feeling so hopeless and sad that you're thinking of hurting yourself, or if you feel that your health or life are in danger, you should call 911 immediately. Even if you're not certain whether or not you're in an emergency situation, just the fact that you're unsure probably means you should call. It never hurts to be too safe, but it can hurt if you don't protect yourself. What happens when you call? A person who works the switchboard answers the phone and asks you why you're calling. After you tell the person how you're feeling, police officers and paramedics come to where you are and escort you to a hospital emergency room. The next section tells you what happens next.

**HOSPITAL EMERGENCY ROOM:** When you think of a hospital emergency room (E.R.), you probably picture a place where people go for a broken leg or if they're having a heart attack. But people also go to an E.R. if they're feeling emotionally out of control or in danger. You can walk into any hospital E.R. and somebody will help you, or you can ask the police to bring you. Most hospitals have special E.R.s just for kids. Once you're there, a counselor will talk to you about what you're feeling and why, and determine the best way for you to stay safe. You might end up going home to have your family take extra special care of you while you see a therapist. Or you might end up staying in the hospital under the supervision of professionals for one or more nights.

## Just Hanging On

Sometimes a girl feels so frightened and hopeless that she considers taking her own life. Usually the girl doesn't really want to die, she just desperately needs things to change. When she is stopped from harming herself, she generally feels incredibly relieved that she was prevented from doing something that she could never take back. She's also grateful to receive assistance in changing what was making her feel so miserable and in learning that she can be happy again. So if you're thinking about hurting yourself, call 911 right now or a hotline number, or get an adult you trust to take you to a hospital E.R. I want you to stay alive and healthy, and get help to feel happy and hopeful.

### ACTION: Reaching Out

1. **Act Now:** If you're considering contacting somebody for help but are still not sure, take a deep breath and let it out. Then, dial a number, go to a website, or visit your school counselor. Be assured that reaching out for help is the most mature move you can make. Help is just around the corner.

2. **Use the Resources Listed in This Book:** Refer to the lists of resources at the end of each chapter. If you can't quite find the perfect listing, call a related one and ask them to refer you.

3. **Learning More About the Process:**

a. **Talk with somebody you know who's been to counseling:** Ask the person what it was like.

b. **Rent a movie:** Watch *Ordinary People* and *Good Will Hunting*—two excellent films that give you a sense of what therapy might be like and how different therapists have very different styles.

4. **If You Still Have Pressing Unanswered Questions:** Please send them my way via my website *The-GirlsGuides.com*, where I'll post questions and answers.

Taking the first step is always the hardest. I know you have the strength to ask for help. With so many people out there to assist you, you will be able to find comfort and help in no time. If you're feeling happy in your life now, then keep in mind that this chapter and the book's resources are here for you when and if you need them. I'm not ready to say good-bye to you quite yet. Turn the page. . . .

# Check Out These Resources

## Phone Numbers

Kid Save Hotline (Suicide Hotline)
1 (800) 543-7283 (24-hours: Crisis intervention and referrals.)

National Runaway Switchboard
1 (800) 621-4000 (24-hours: Even though they specialize in issues of running away, you can call them anytime with any problem you might have.)

Action—A Parent and Teen Support Line
1 (800) FOR-TEEN or (800) 367-8336) (24 hours: Call them with any problem on your mind.)

Youth Line
1-800-246-4646 (24 hours)

International Child Abuse Network—Yes ICAN
(888) 224-4226 (Regular weekday hours for referrals.)

*http://www.yesican.org*: Chat with girls struggling with similar issues; a trained counselor facilitates the discussion.

*http://www.acf.dhhs.gov/programs/cb/rpt_abu.htm*: Provides child abuse hotlines, listed by state.

## Books

Pipher, Mary. *Reviving Ophelia: Saving the Selves of Adolescent Girls.* New York: Ballantine Books, 1995.
Shandler, Sara. *Ophelia Speaks: Adolescent Girls Write About Their Search for Self.* New York: HarperCollins, 1999.

# Conclusion

# Good-bye For Now...

Are you a body blues resister yet? It can take a while for new confidences to build and for experiments in health to become healthy habits. Let me know if the people in your life start calling you the Energizer. While I'm dance-skating nonstop for three to five hours, skaters are constantly rolling up to me and saying, "Hey, you're just like that Energizer bunny who keeps going and going." Then they'll jokingly look for my battery pack, and when they don't find it, they ask, "What's your energizing secret?" When I tell them it's just that I take good care of my body, they seem a little disappointed, like they wanted me to hand them a magic pill. Now you know my secrets better than anybody: a down-to-earth recipe for feeling healthy and good about yourself. Remember, you are a mover and a shaker with boundless energy and potential.

In the past, females were the models for paintings, statues, and photographs. Today, we're the painters, sculptors, and photographers. Adult females used to be defined mostly by how they looked on the outside, how many children they had, and what their husbands did. Now women, like men, can be distinguished from each other by their interests and professions—by what they are on the inside. A college-age friend of mine reports that when she was in preschool, all the mothers were doctors. She remembers that one day at leaving time, a little boy ran over to his mother and asked, "Mommy, Mommy, can boys be doctors too?" You are living on the cutting edge of history. You are free to feel the strength, beauty, and grace of your body while also exploring the power of your mind.

> In ancient Greece, marriage was considered such an important aspect of a woman's identity that she counted her age from the date of her wedding, not from the day she was born.

Exercise your right to independent thinking and let me know what you thought of this book—what you found helpful and what you didn't. Is there anything important that I left out? Maybe you have your own resister tips you'd like to offer girls—send them to me and I can post them for others. Let me know what you want the topic of my next book to be, whether it be friendship, fashion, boys, or anything else that gets your head spinning with confusion. So visit me at *www.TheGirlsGuides.com*, and let me know what's on your mind. You can even sneak a peek at my dance-skating and watch me shoot a basketball; any tips on how I can improve my shooting form will be very welcome!

So until we meet again on the Web, keep on groovin'. . . .

# Endnotes

1 Heiman, *US Report: The Incredible Shrinking Woman* (read online).
2 Immell, *Contemporary Issues Companion: Eating Disorders*, p. 65.
3 Heiman, *US Report: The Incredible Shrinking Woman* (read online).
4 Sneddon, *Body Image: A Reality Check (Issues in Focus)*, p. 18.
5 Hamm, *Go for the Goal*, pp. 3–4.
6 Blais, *In These Girls Hope Is a Muscle*, p. 113.
7 Hamm, *Go for the Goal*, p. 6.
8 Blais, *In These Girls Hope Is a Muscle*, p. 234.
9 Bode, *Food Fight: A Guide to Eating Disorders for Preteens and Their Parents*, p. 85.
10 Immell, *Contemporary Issues Companion: Eating Disorders*, p. 144.
11 Sneddon, *Body Image: A Reality Check (Issues in Focus)*, p. 43.
12 Immell, *Contemporary Issues Companion: Eating Disorders*, pp. 143–144.
13 Kaminker, *Exercise Addiction: When Fitness Becomes an Obsession (The Teen Health Library of Eating Disorder Prevention)*, p. 32.
14 Bode, *Food Fight: A Guide to Eating Disorders for Preteens and Their Parents*, pp. 43–44.

15 Bode, *Food Fight: A Guide to Eating Disorders for Preteens and Their Parents*, p. 71.

16 Kaminker, *Exercise Addiction: When Fitness Becomes an Obsession (The Teen Health Library of Eating Disorder Prevention)*, p. 31.

17 Chiu, *Eating Disorder: Survivors Tell Their Stories (The Teen Health Library of Eating Disorder Prevention)*, p. 39.

18 Chiu, *Eating Disorder: Survivors Tell Their Stories (The Teen Health Library of Eating Disorder Prevention)*, p. 47.

19 Chiu, *Eating Disorder: Survivors Tell Their Stories (The Teen Health Library of Eating Disorder Prevention)*, p. 45.

20 Immell, *Contemporary Issues Companion: Eating Disorders*, p. 168.

21 Kaminker, *Exercise Addiction: When Fitness Becomes an Obsession (The Teen Health Library of Eating Disorder Prevention)*, p. 31.

22 Chiu, *Eating Disorder: Survivors Tell Their Stories (The Teen Health Library of Eating Disorder Prevention)*, p. 19.

23 Kaminker, *Exercise Addiction: When Fitness Becomes an Obsession (The Teen Health Library of Eating Disorder Prevention)*, p. 31.

24 Bode, *Food Fight: A Guide to Eating Disorders for Preteens and Their Parents*, p. 49.

25 Bode, *Food Fight: A Guide to Eating Disorders for Preteens and Their Parents*, p. 50.

26 Bode, *Food Fight: A Guide to Eating Disorders for Preteens and Their Parents*, p. 50.

27 Bode, *Food Fight: A Guide to Eating Disorders for Preteens and Their Parents*, p. 61.

28 Shandler, *Ophelia Speaks: Adolescent Girls Write About Their Search for Self*, p. 25.

29 Bode, *Food Fight: A Guide to Eating Disorders for Preteens and Their Parents*, p. 72.

# Bibliography

*Annual Editions: Drugs, Society & Behavior 99/00.* 14th ed. An Instructor's Resource Guide. Guilford, Connecticut: Dushkin/McGraw-Hill, 1999.

Asimov, Isaac. *Isaac Asimov's Book of Facts.* New York: Random House Value Publishing, Inc., 1997.

Barrett, CeCe. *The Dangers of Diet Drugs and Other Weight-Loss Products (The Teen Health Library of Eating Disorder Prevention).* New York: The Rosen Publishing Group, Inc., 1999.

Bell, Ruth. *Changing Bodies, Changing Lives: A Book for Teens on Sex and Relationships.* New York: Times Books, Random House, 1998.

Berg, Eric. *Anorexia: Am I at Risk? A Food and Feelings Checklist.* Santa Cruz: ETR Associates, 1997.

——*Bulimia: Am I at Risk? A Food and Feelings Checklist.* Santa Cruz: ETR Associates, 1997.

——*Food and Feelings.* Santa Cruz: ETR Associates, 1992.

——*Teens and Marijuana: Get Real About Pot!* Santa Cruz: ETR Associates, 1999.

*Beyond Nutrition: Eating for Health.* Lake Zurich, Illinois: The Learning Seed, 1999. (video, 22 mins.)

Bidwell, Andrea. *Focus on Fat Food Lab.* Owatonna, Minneapolis: Pineapple Appeal/Low-Fat Express/Learning Zone (no date).

Blais, Madeline. *In These Girls Hope Is a Muscle.* New York: Atlantic Monthly Press, 1995.

Bode, Janet. *Food Fight: A Guide to Eating Disorders for*

*Preteens and Their Parents.* New York: Aladdin Paperbacks, Simon & Schuster, 1997.

Brody, Jane E. "New Respect for the Nap, A Pause That Refreshes." *New York Times* 4 Jan. 2000.

Brooke, James. "Even Quebec Gets Tough on Smoking." *New York Times* 25 Jan. 2000: F8.

Brumberg, Joan Jacobs. *The Body Project: An Intimate History of American Girls.* New York: Random House, 1997.

Chiu, Christina. *Eating Disorder: Survivors Tell Their Stories (The Teen Health Library of Eating Disorder Prevention).* New York: The Rosen Publishing Group, Inc., 1998.

*Choose to Refuse: Saying No and Keeping Your Friends.* Exec. Prod. Anson W. Schloat. Human Relations Media, Inc., 1993. (video, 25 min. approx.)

Copeland, Larry J., M.D. *Textbook of Gynecology.* Philadelphia: W.B. Saunders Company, 1993.

Davis, Brangien. *What's Real, What's Ideal: Overcoming a Negative Body Image (The Teen Health Library of Eating Disorder Prevention).* New York: The Rosen Publishing Group, Inc., 1999.

Dixon, Monica A., MS, RD. *Fun'tastic Nutrition Education Ideas. Innovative teaching techniques for secondary students.* Owatonna, Minnesota: Pineapple Appeal/Low-Fat Express/Learning Zone, 1995 (revised).

Drohan, Michele Ingber. *Weight-Loss Programs: Weighing the Risks and Realities (The Teen Health Library of Eating Disorder Prevention).* New York: The Rosen Publishing Group, Inc., 1998.

Duyff, Roberta Larson, MS, RD, CFCS. *The American Dietetic Association's Complete Food & Nutrition Guide.* Minneapolis: Chronimed Publishing, 1996.

ETR Associates. *Incredible Food Facts.* Santa Cruz: ETR Associates, 1998.

*Fad Diets: The Weight Loss Merry-Go-Round.* Bloomington, Illinois: Meridian education corporation. (video, 16 mins.)

*The Fast Food Caper: What's In It For You.* Cambridge Career Products. Charleston, West Virginia: Cambridge Research Group, Ltd., 1990. (video, 30 mins.)

Fellner, Jane, MD, ABFP. *Help on the Way: Bulimia.* Santa Cruz: ETR Associates, 1996.

*Fit or Fat for the 90's.* Perf. Covert Bailey. Atlanta, Georgia: KVIE, Inc. (program), Turner Home Entertainment (artwork & design), PBS Home Video, 1991, 1994. (Video, 77 mins.)

Flaherty, Julie. "Perk du Jour: A Well-Stocked Kitchen." *New York Times* 12 Jan. 2000: G1.

Garofalo, Robert, M.D. "Sexual Orientation and Risk of Suicide Attempts Among a Representative Sample of Youth." *Pediatric and Adolescent Medicine* 153. May 1999: 487.

*The Girls Project: Girls Empowering Girls. A training workbook for girls, their teachers, sisters, moms, aunts and other friends.* New York: Institute for Labor & the Community (ILC), 1998.

Glass, George. *Drugs and Fitting In (The Drug Abuse Prevention Library).* New York: The Rosen Publishing Group, Inc., 1998.

Grabish, Beatrice R. *Drugs and Your Brain (The Drug Abuse Prevention Library).* New York: The Rosen Publishing Group, Inc., 1998.

Grady, Denise. "Genetic Damage in Young Smokers Is Linked to Lung Cancer." *New York Times* 7 Apr. 1999: A17.

Grosshandler, Janet. *Drugs and the Law (The Drug Abuse Prevention Library).* New York: The Rosen Publishing Group, Inc., 1993.

Hamm, Mia. *Go for the Goal: A Champion's Guide to Winning in Soccer and Life.* New York: HarperCollins, 1999.

Hanan, Jessica. *When Someone You Love Is Addicted (The Drug Abuse Prevention Library).* New York: The Rosen Publishing Group, Inc., 1990.

*Healthy Snacking.* Owatonna, Minnesota: Pineapple Appeal/Low-Fat Express/Learning Zone (no date).

Heiman, J.D. *US Magazine*: *The Incredible Shrinking Woman,* September 1999.

"Hemp Foods: All the Nutrition, Without the High." *Environmental Nutrition* Jan. 2000: 3.

Hemphill, Clara. "A Cure for Acne, a Treatment for Angst." *New York Times* 29 Feb. 2000: F1+.

Hiatt, Jane. *Alcohol Self-Test.* Santa Cruz: ETR Associates, 1997.

Immell, Myra H., ed. *Contemporary Issues Companion: Eating Disorders.* San Diego: Greenhaven Press, Inc., 1999.

Jacobson, Michael F., Ph.D., and Sarah Fritschner. *The Completely Revised and Updated Fast-Food Guide.* 2nd ed. New York: Workman Publishing, 1991.

Jukes, Mavis. *It's A Girl Thing: How to Stay Healthy, Safe, and in Charge.* New York: Alfred A. Knopf, 1997.

Kaminker, Laura. *Exercise Addiction: When Fitness Becomes an Obsession (The Teen Health Library of Eating Disorder Prevention).* New York: The Rosen Publishing Group, Inc., 1998.

Lang, Alan R., Ph. D. *Alcohol: Teenage Drinking (The Encyclopedia of Psychoactive Drugs).* New York, Philadelphia: Chelsea House Publishers, 1992 (revised).

Langer, Micheal B. Langer. *Drugs and the Pressure to be Perfect (The Drug Abuse Prevention Library).* New York: The Rosen Publishing Group, Inc., 1998.

Lawrance, Lynette K., Ph.D. *The Fats of Life.* Santa Cruz: ETR Associates, 1997.

Lee, Richard S., and Mary Price. *Caffeine and Nicotine (The Drug Abuse Prevention Library).* New York: The Rosen Publishing Group, Inc., 1998.

Louis, David. *2201 Fascinating Facts.* New York: Random House Value Publishing, Inc., The Ridge Press, Inc., and Crown Publishers, Inc., 1983.

Madaras, Lynda, and Area Madaras. *The What's Happening to My Body? Book for Girls.* New York: Newmarket Press, 1987.

Maharg, Ruth, MA, MPH. *Real World Drinking*. Santa Cruz: ETR Associates, 1998.

————*Real World Marijuana*. Santa Cruz: ETR Associates, 1998.

————*Real World Smoking*. Santa Cruz: ETR Associates, 1998.

McMillan, Daniel. *Teen Smoking: Understanding the Risk (Issues in Focus)*. Springfield, New Jersey: Enslow Publishers, Inc., 1998.

Monk, Arlene, and Nancy Cooper. *Convenience Food Facts: A Quick Guide for Choosing Healthy Brand-Name Foods in Every Aisle of the Supermarket*. 4th ed. Minneapolis: IDC Publishing, 1997.

Moskowitz, Eva. *The Therapeutic Gospel*. Baltimore: Johns Hopkins Press, 2000.

Mueller, Melinda M., MS. *Marijuana*. Santa Cruz: ETR Associates, 1996.

Nagourney, Eric. "For Some, Vegan Diet Relieves PMS." *New York Times* 15 Feb. 2000.

————"Trouble for Women in the Mess Hall." *New York Times* 18 Jan. 2000.

Ornish, Dean, MD. *Eat More, Weigh Less*. New York: HarperCollins Publishers, 1993.

Owens, Daryl E. "Boy Crazy!: Cards are a bad idea, experts say." *Baltimore Sun* 12 Mar. 2000: 1N+.

Parrott, Andy C. "Does Cigarette Smoking Cause Stress?" *American Psychologist* 54.10. Oct. 1999.

Peterson, Pamela Gilbeau, Ph.D. *About Marijuana*. Santa Cruz: ETR Associates, 1990.

————*Drug Facts*. Santa Cruz: ETR Associates, 1990.

————*Tobacco Facts*. Santa Cruz: ETR Associates, 1999.

Piper, Watty. *The Little Engine That Could*. New York: Platt & Munk, 1961, c 1930.

Pringle, Lawrence. *Drinking: A Risky Business*. New York: Morrow Junior Books, 1997.

Proudfoot, Linda. *Bodies: Incredible Facts*. Santa Cruz: ETR Associates, 1998.

————*Incredible Dieting Facts.* Santa Cruz: ETR Associates, 1999.

Quakenbush, Marcia, MS, MFCC, CHES. *Eating Well: What's In It for Me?* Santa Cruz: ETR Associates, 1999.

Rashbaum, William K. "Drug Experts Report a Boom in Ecstasy Use." *New York Times* 26 Feb. 2000: B1.

Robinson, Thomas N., M.D. "Reducing Children's Television Viewing to Prevent Obesity: A Randomized Controlled Trial." *Journal of the American Medical Association* 282. 27 Oct. 1999: 1561.

Rosenthal, Elisabeth. "China's Chic Waistline: Convex to Concave." *New York Times* 9 Dec. 1999: A1+.

Ross, Karen, LCSW. *Eating Disorders.* Santa Cruz: ETR Associates, 1996.

Salter, Charles A. *The Nutrition-Fitness Link: A Teen Nutrition Book.* Brookfield, Connecticut: The Millbrook Press, 1993.

Schaefer, Valorie L. *The Care and Keeping of You: The Body Book for Girls (American Girl Library Series).* Middleton, Wisconsin: Pleasant Company Publications, 1998.

Schneider, Max A., M.D. *Addiction.* Santa Cruz: ETR Associates, 1992.

*Selling Addiction: A Workshop Kit on Tobacco and Alcohol Advertising: Consumer Seduction.* Perf. Michael Learned. Los Angeles, California: Scott Newman Center, 1992. (video)

*Selling Addiction: A Workshop Kit on Tobacco and Alcohol Advertising: Selling Addiction: Video Segments.* Perf. Michael Learned. Los Angeles, California: Center for Media and Values, 1992. (video)

Shandler, Sara. *Ophelia Speaks: Adolescent Girls Write About Their Search for Self.* New York: HarperCollins, 1999.

Sneddon, Pamela Shires. *Body Image: A Reality Check (Issues in Focus).* Springfield, New Jersey: Enslow Publishers, Inc., 1999.

Stacy, Lori Moore. *Beautiful You! The All About You Guide to Looking and Feeling Your Best.* New York: Scholastic Inc., 1999.

Stang, Jamie, Ph.D. *Preventing Eating Disorders.* Owatonna, Minnesota: Learning Zone Express (no date).

Stearns, Peter N. *Fat History: Bodies and Beauty in the Modern West.* New York: New York University, 1997.

Van Natta Jr., Don. "Drug Office Will End Its Scrutiny of TV Scripts." *New York Times* 20 Jan. 2000.

Walsh, Brian J. *Teens and Alcohol (Social Issues Series).* US: The Center for Learning, 1998.

Wilson, Hugh T., Ph.D., ed. *Annual Editions: Drugs, Society & Behavior 99/00.* 14th ed. Guilford, Connecticut: Dushkin/McGraw-Hill, 1999.

Wren, Christopher S. "More Teenagers Disapprove of Drug Use, Survey Finds." *New York Times* 22 Nov. 1999.

Yoon, Carol Kaesuk. "Of Beasts, Behavior and the Size of Litters." *New York Times* 19 Oct. 1999: F3.